NUTRITIONAL
SOLUTIONS FOR
88 CONDITIONS

Correct the Causes

DAVID ROWLAND

BALBOA.
PRESS
A DIVISION OF HAY HOUSE

Balboa Press books may be ordered through booksellers or by contacting:

Balboa Press
A Division of Hay House
1663 Liberty Drive
Bloomington, IN 47403
www.balboapress.com
1 (877) 407-4847

Print information available on the last page.

ISBN: 978-1-5043-6978-7 (sc)
ISBN: 978-1-5043-6979-4 (e)

Balboa Press rev. date: 12/16/2016

CONTENTS

FOREWORD

by **Bryce Wylde**, B.Sc., DHMHS

Associate Medical Director at P3 Health, City TV Health Expert, Medical Advisor Dr. OZ show

I grew up eating a vegetarian diet but intuitively felt I may have been missing something. I began to include meat, but still felt my diet was 'off'. I always ensured the meat I ate was organic, a result of humane practices, sustainable, and had minimal environmental impact.

Then, I came across the book, *One's Food is Another's Poison*, by David Rowland; and it dawned on me that the impact nutrition has on our health isn't always about what is deemed healthy versus unhealthy. Keep in mind this was 20 years ago and long before "food sensitivities" were popularized. After reading this eye opening book, it became apparent to me that foods that were considered healthy for the general population could behave like slow poisons in those who are sensitive to them. I was able to identify and get rid of a number of offending foods, and my energy and overall sense of wellness was changed forever.

Later on, over the course of my graduate program, I came across another of David Rowland's books, *THE NUTRITIONAL BYPASS: Reverse Atherosclerosis Without Surgery*. This was also a game changer and further substantiated what I was already coming to learn - that food has a profound impact on our health. Nutrition impacts every single organ and every single cell in our body. We can prevent disease onset using nutrition, but what's more is we can reverse many diseases using select diet and nutrients.

Optimal nutrition is irrefutably the cornerstone of good health. In fact, the idea is nearly as old as recorded history. You have seen or at least heard Hippocrates' famous quote: *"Let food be thy medicine and let medicine be thy food"*.

More than 1500 years later, in about 1920, the very popular phrase "you are what you eat" was first coined by nutritionist Victor Lindlahr. He was a strong believer in the idea that food controls health. *"Ninety per cent of the diseases known to man are caused by cheap foodstuffs."* wrote Lindlahr. This view has gained many adherents in the last century.

But to this very day across North America, the pharmaceutical industry maintains its control; and many conventionally trained doctors remain dismissive of nutritional therapies. Are doctors ready to think outside the operatory or past the pillbox? Conventional practitioners who are dismissive about the power of food and nutrients in health and disease quite simply have their heads buried in the sand.

It is nearly impossible to ignore the powerful scientific evidence, such as the Mediterranean diet shown to reduce the incidence of major cardiovascular events by 30%, or that elemental diets can serve as treatment for inflammatory bowel disease (often better than drug therapy), and the multiple studies examining the relationship between the over consumption of fast food and animal products (including dairy) and chronic illnesses such as coronary heart disease, diabetes, breast cancer, prostate cancer, and bowel cancer.

In spite of all the evidence, a significant nutrition gap remains in North America – a serious disconnect between how patients and doctors perceive diet. From fad diets to unsubstantiated supplements there are so many "nutritional therapies" out there, so many programs with so many claims, and so little science to back them up that it's no wonder that it's hard for sound nutritional therapies to break through. That is...until now.

David Rowland is the foremost expert in holistic nutrition, author of 12 highly acclaimed health publications, innovator and publisher of Nutritiapedia®, creator of Nutri-Body® assessment, founder of the Canadian Nutrition Institute and the Edison Institute of Nutrition. Rowland has cut through the noise and offers a plethora of no-nonsense nutritional solutions in this - his latest work, ***NUTRITIONAL SOLUTIONS FOR 88 CONDITIONS: Correct the Causes***.

This book is the most relevant, useful and comprehensive compilation of contemporary holistic nutrition information I have read to date. In these pages you will find all of David Rowland's best research and clinical experience complete with new and innovative programs to naturally address - and in many cases prevent disease altogether.

It will quickly become apparent that David Rowland is no ordinary nutritionist and that he comes with many decades of experience. He is a trailblazer and trendsetter but simultaneously uninterested in medical buzz terms or fads. Long before organics were trending, he was teaching us about the impact of pesticides and soil depletion. Prior to what has become common knowledge linking nutrition and our genes, he was one of the first to effectively address nutritional and biochemical individuality. Well before mainstream began picking up on the importance of detoxification, or acknowledging the incidence of gluten sensitivity, or appreciating the legitimacy of leaky gut syndrome, the epidemic of inflammation underlying the majority of heart disease, or the infamous candida connection now linked to many common health problems, Rowland was providing safe and effective holistic nutritional solutions for these and hundreds of other conditions. He has always been steadfast in upholding and teaching the fundamentals of holistic nutrition and micronutrient supplementation but goes beyond to steer clear of the junk in order to provide you with sensible, easy to understand, and actionable solutions to your health concerns.

Whether your goal is to maintain ideal weight, gain energy, boost your immune system and prevent infection, manage your blood sugar or improve your eyesight, enhance your mental health or prevent osteoporosis, by reading this book you will gain newfound insights into optimizing your health. Among other things, this work sheds light on the cholesterol myth and how to unplug your arteries and maintain your heart health for life. You will augment your perspective on preventing cancer and living a longer more satisfying existence.

The English professor, farmer, novelist and poet, Wendell Berry, astutely noted, *"People are fed by the food industry, which pays no attention to health and are treated by the health industry, which pays no attention to food"*. David Rowland has made it his calling to bring attention to the power of self-healing and help bridge the gap between nutrition and health.

Nutritional Solutions for 88 Conditions is incisive and illuminating. There is something for everyone in this book. If you believe your health is an investment and not an expense, turn the page!

OVERVIEW

*"There are many paths to the top of the mountain,
and the view is always the same."*

-Chinese proverb

There are many ways to overcome disease, and all of them require giving the body whatever it needs to do its own self-healing. The therapeutic perspective I am about to share with you is time proven for correcting the causes of many degenerative conditions. That is not to say that this is the only nutritional modality that works. It is simply the one with which I am most familiar, having witnessed countless successes in my 38 years of experience with it.

The only sure way to overcome any health challenge is to correct its cause. The emphasis of this book is thus on understanding nutritional biochemistry and what interferes with its optimal functioning. Once cause and effect are understood, then the solutions are obvious.

RESULTS

The principles in this book can enable you to achieve results that are not generally believed possible. Thousands of others have done just that. In reviewing a sample of 200 "thank you" letters, I found that almost half of the writers had experienced significant cardiovascular benefits – including removing arterial plaque, avoiding bypass surgery, avoiding amputation, getting rid of angina, lowering cholesterol, and lowering blood pressure.

Next frequently mentioned in these letters was improved digestion for which other methods had failed – followed by thyroid function restored without resort to pharmaceuticals – followed by the remission of five different kinds of cancer. Other conditions completely overcome included enlarged prostate, adrenal weakness, cataracts, arthritis, attention deficit disorder (ADD), seizures, and heavy metal toxicity. A surprising number of writers also reported less dependence on insulin for controlling their diabetes.

HOLISTIC NUTRITION

Holism is the theory that certain wholes are greater than the sum of their parts. This is most certainly true with respect to nutrition. It is often misleading to look for a single deficiency as a possible cause for any condition. Nutrients are synergistic. A number of metaphors apply:

- Nutrition is like a chain in which all of the links have to be strong. If only one or two essential nutrients are lacking, the health of the entire body can suffer.
- Nutrition is teamwork. Lack of performance from one team member reduces the output for the entire team.
- Nutrition is like an orchestra, with some nutrients carrying the melody and others the harmony.

For example, your body could have a shortage of three nutrients but not be able to utilize those three fully unless it also has an abundance of four other nutrients. Unless you provide all seven factors in suitable proportions, you may not be able to achieve the results you desire.

DIVERSITY

There is no one diet that is ideal for everyone. Over centuries, humans have adapted to whatever natural food sources are available. Our paleolithic ancestors thrived on wild game, organ meats, greens, nuts, and roots. The Inuit thrived on meat, fish, blubber, and birds – the Maasai on milk, blood and meat – the Iroquois on corn, beans, and squash – plains tribes on bison, large and small game, and berries – the Aztecs on corn, beans, avocadoes, sweet potatoes, peppers, and tomatoes – the Japanese on fish, seaweed, tofu, and vegetables - Hindus on lentils, beans, cottage cheese, and ghee – and Mediterranean countries on lean meats, fish, eggs, cheese, yogurt, vegetables, fruits, and olive oil.

As diverse as the above traditional diets are, they all have two things in common: (1) sufficiently high protein content, and (2) stable fats. Failure to provide these two critical essentials in our modern diets causes many degenerative conditions to which our ancestors were immune.

PROTEIN

The word, protein, comes to us from Greek that translates as "of first importance". The body needs protein to make DNA, hormones, enzymes, antibodies, hemoglobin (to carry oxygen in the blood), myoglobin and elastin (for muscle tissues), collagen (for skin, tendons, cartilage, bones, joints), and keratin (for hair and nails).

When all of the uses of protein are considered, most adults probably require more than the daily recommended intake (DRI) of 0.36 grams per pound of bodyweight – which figure is based on structural requirements and overlooks the role of protein in making hormones, enzymes, and antibodies. A safer level of protein intake is 60 grams per day for women, and 80 grams per day for men, and pregnant or lactating women (regardless of bodyweight in each case).

Inadequate protein intake causes premature aging, hormonal imbalances, immune weakness, fluid retention (edema), anemia, cataracts, muscle wasting, low resistance to stress, hair loss in women, and loss of menstrual flow (amenorrhea). [*As a visual reference: 20 grams of meat protein is about the size of a deck of playing cards.*]

We have animal bodies that require proteins that are as complete in their amino acid structure as are foods of animal origin (e.g., meat, fish, eggs, cheese). To get complete protein from plant sources, we have to combine legumes plus grains at every meal (e.g., beans + corn, lentils + rice, chickpeas + whole wheat). The one exception to this food combining rule is soy/tofu, which is very close to the amino acid structure of meat.

STABLE FATS

All of the traditional diets from every culture include only stable fats – such as the fat on meat, fish oils, avocadoes, coconut oil, olive oil, or butter. None of these diets include polyunsaturated oils, which are chemically unstable and readily break down in the body to form damaging free radicals.

Human milk contains a saturated fat (palmitic acid) and a monounsaturated fat (oleic acid), both of which are chemically stable. Nature is telling us that these are the safe fats to consume.

Fats are required (a) as a backup energy source when carbohydrates run out, (b) to absorb and distribute vitamins A, D, E and K, (c) to help maintain core body temperature, (d) to cushion internal organs, (e) to make prostaglandins (intermediate hormone-like substances), (f) to regulate the production of sex hormones, and last but not least (g) to maintain the integrity of cellular membranes, an important immune function.

Cellular membranes that contain a high percentage of polyunsaturates become vulnerable to destruction by free radicals and invasion by viruses. Whenever our ancestors consumed polyunsaturates, it was in moderation and as an integral part of whole nuts and seeds, nature's protective packaging. The temptation with extracted polyunsaturated oils is to consume them to excess.

Fish oils provide the omega-3 fatty acids, DHA and EPA. DHA (docosahexanoic acid) is a structural component of the brain and is responsible the saying, "fish is brain food". EPA (eicosapentanoic acid) is a precursor to prostaglandin-3, which prevents blood platelets from sticking together.

HEALTHY DIETS

There are a number of very different approaches that are promoted as the one best way to eat – various versions of omnivorous, lacto-ovo-vegetarian, vegetarian plus fish, and total vegetarian (vegan) diets. What they all have in common is the total absence of refined sugars, refined flour, processed foods, and hydrogenated fats. If you simply stop consuming these artificial foods, then no matter how else you eat can be very healthy for you.

Dietary fiber is critical for healthy elimination and is provided only by the cell walls of plants. The more animal protein that is consumed, the more it needs to counterbalanced with similar amounts of vegetables, whole grains, and fruits.

Vitamin B-12 and heme iron are found only in foods of animal origin. The higher the vegetarian content of a diet, the more need there is to supplement with B-12 and ferrous fumarate (an organic plant source of iron).

Vegan diets require vigilance to ensure adequate protein intake. If your only source of protein is plant based, then at every meal you need to combine legumes (e.g., beans, peas, lentils, chickpeas) with grains (e.g., rice, corn, whole wheat) in the ratio of 1:3 (one part legume to three parts grain). The only time this protein combining can be relaxed is if the meal contains a substantial amount of soy, preferably as tofu.

Agricultural soils are deficient in iodine, selenium, and zinc. If these minerals are not in the soil, they are also not in the plants, which cannot pass them on to the animals that eat the plants. Regardless of the composition of one's diet, it makes sense to take supplements of at least these three minerals.

THERAPEUTIC DIETS

Extreme diets that can help to restore health are not necessarily capable of maintaining long term health. The Pritikin, McDougall, and Ornish plans are examples of low fat, high starch, low protein diets intended to reduce one's risk of cardiovascular disease. These are therapeutic diets that can provide immediate short term benefits, but are incapable of sustaining long term optimal health.

When total fat intake is restricted to 10 percent of total calories, this puts the body into a starvation mode whereby it has to cannibalize the deposits in arteries in order to get enough fats for survival. Once the arterial fats are used up, however, the intake of dietary fats is incapable of maintaining the integrity of cellular membranes. The result is clear arteries at the expense of an increased risk for cancer. For long term maintenance, one needs to consume at least 22 percent of calories in the form of stable fats.

All of the above low fat diets are also too low in quality protein for long term maintenance. After two years on a low protein diet, one tends to age rapidly, to become generally weak, to handle stress poorly, and to be vulnerable to mood swings, depression, nervousness, agitation, and cataracts.

The redeeming feature of low-fat, low-protein diets is that they are so severe that hardly anyone can stay on them for any length of time. Starving the body of fats and proteins is a time bomb waiting to go off, and most people can sense this before it is too late. Either they quit the program entirely, modify it to be more sensible, or succumb to the frequent eating binges the body induces to get what it desperately needs.

FOOD SUPPLEMENTS

Throughout history, humans have been getting their vitamin C and antioxidants from fruits and berries, neither of which contribute any protein or fats to the diet. In this sense, fruits/berries serve as food supplements. We humans have a high need for vitamin C, which is scarce in nature and found mainly in sweet tasting plants. Our affinity for sweets is nature's way of ensuring that we get enough vitamin C.

Holistic food supplementation requires making sure that the body has an abundance of everything needed for optimal functioning. Give the body a banquet of all the nutrients it could possibly require, and it fills up on what it needs and ignores that which it already has.

The emphasis in holistic nutrition is on providing the essentials that the body cannot produce itself, then letting the body take it from there. Essential amino acids and essential fatty acids are most efficiently provided by a diet that deliberately includes them. If one wishes to build superior health (and not merely the absence of disease), then it is also necessary to take a broad spectrum of vitamin and mineral supplements. A bonus of this approach is that if your body has all of the vitamins and minerals it needs, it can make all of the intermediate nutrients it requires (e.g., coenzyme Q_{10}, gamma linolenic acid, glutathione).

The quantities of supplementary nutrients required to build and maintain optimal health are significantly higher than recommended daily allowances (RDAs) suggest. When you give your body a suitably potent combination of 26 vitamins and minerals, the first thing you will notice is that bodily discomforts and inconveniences tend to disappear – subtle things you have been enduring, not realizing that faulty nutrition could be involved. Full blown deficiency disorders and a number of degenerative conditions also disappear when on an optimal supplement program. Any that do not fade away on their own will require extra therapeutic measures.

Nutritional therapy works as an adjunct to optimal nutrition, rather than as a substitute for it. Taking only those supplements intended to improve a specific condition is a fragmented approach that works for something that requires immediate attention, but does nothing to prevent chronic underlying issues from becoming full blown conditions further down the road. Often, the fragmented approach may be ameliorating symptoms rather than correcting causes.

Therapeutic nutrition requires providing an orchestrated blend of all of the essential nutrients that treat the specific condition in question – including select vitamins and/or minerals, and sometimes key amino acids (e.g., cysteine, tyrosine, methionine). Sometimes select herbs may be added, if they provide synergistic factors. In some cases, homeopathic remedies may also be used to help the body detoxify from specific threats.

BIOCHEMICAL INDIVIDUALITY

"It is more important to know the person who has the condition than it is to know what condition the person has." - Hippocrates

Biologically, we are created unequal. We have different faces, fingerprints, and voices. On the inside, we are just as different. Roger Williams was a researcher who discovered significant anatomical and physiological variations from person to person. He coined the term "biochemical individuality" to describe this phenomenon. Internal organs vary in size, structure, and efficiency – which means that they also have varying requirements for specific nutrients.

Some of us are born with metabolic weaknesses that require extra nutritional attention. The ability to digest, absorb, and assimilate nutrients varies widely. Having enough of a given nutrient in our diet is not sufficient; we also have to ensure that it gets to the cells that need it. A surprising number of people have been found to require from 20 to 40 times the amount of a particular vitamin than most others do. Stressful lifestyles increase the demands for key nutrients.

A "one size fits all" nutritional approach is of limited value. There is no one diet that is ideal for everyone. Neither is there any nutritional remedy that works for everyone. Textbook theories do not always apply to individuals. Neither do studies or statistics. Of what value to you is it to know that a particular piece of nutritional advice applies to 80 percent of the population if you happen to be in the 20 percent to whom it does not?

Linus Pauling coined the term, orthomolecular, to mean "the right molecule in the right amounts". There is an optimum nutritional environment in the body, and disease reflect deficiencies in this environment. The goal of orthomolecular medicine is to correct imbalances and deficiencies based on individual biochemistry. Easier said than done, if one assumes that every person with the same condition has the identical nutritional environment.

Blood tests measure many things, but they cannot tell the whole story – and sometimes they are misleading. Why? Because the blood strives to maintain a state of normalcy, and will do so right up to the point of death. It maintains this homeostasis at the expense of other tissues in the body. Examples:

- Blood calcium levels may be normal even during osteoporosis; the blood needs calcium so badly that it may rob bones to get it.
- Blood levels of vitamin B-12 may be normal, even when there is not enough in cerebrospinal fluid.
- Some people, under stress, produce a "mauve factor" which binds vitamin B-6 and zinc, making them unavailable to the rest of the body, even though blood levels of these two nutrients may be normal.
- A vitamin B-12 deficiency can result in misleadingly high levels of folic acid.
- There can be enough thyroid hormones in the blood, but not enough getting to the tissues that need it; these hormones are not primarily transmitted through the bloodstream.

The most reliable way to identify nutritional weaknesses is in their subclinical state, before they show up on laboratory tests. This can be done only by comprehensive analysis of symptoms, such as with my Nutri-Body® system of nutritional assessment that practitioners have been using since 1992. Nutri-Body® analyzes responses to 600 questions pertaining to 65 categories of metabolic imbalances, then ranks these nutritional weaknesses in order of treatment priority. This ranking is based entirely on the person's unique biochemistry and has nothing to do with theories or textbooks, and nothing to do with how others have scored on their tests.

LISTEN TO YOUR BODY

Long before any disease reveals itself, your body lets you know that some things are not working as well as they used to. These messages are usually in the form of pesky little discomforts that we take for granted, not realizing that faulty nutrition may be involved. Energy may be low, there may be mild aches or pains, thinking may be "fuzzy", fingernails break easily, skin is dry, hair lustreless, and so on. These are but a few of the pre-clinical symptoms that the Nutri-Body® method assesses to discover nutritional weaknesses. In this book you will find many more, and what they mean for you.

A number of chapters include lists of symptoms excerpted from the Nutri-Body® questionnaire. Use them to see if you may be heading towards a heart attack or stroke – or to see if you may have low thyroid, weak adrenals, low blood sugar, digestive weakness, gallbladder problems, a candida infection, or a leaky gut.

EVERY DISEASE IS A SYMPTOM

A disease (or condition) is a cluster of symptoms to which we have given a name or label. Once we know what our condition is called, then the usual response is to look for a remedy for the label, giving little or no thought as to cause and effect. This is the "what do I take for my _____" syndrome, which makes outrageous profits for the pharmaceutical industry.

Prescription drugs cannot cure anything. Drugs work by interfering with biochemical pathways. The best that they can do is to relieve symptoms while the body goes about its business of healing itself – which it can do only if you give it what it needs to do the job. Unfortunately, suppressing symptoms (especially pain) provides a false security which encourages one to continue the self-destructive habits which caused the problem, thus making it worse – and also encouraging lifelong dependence on the symptom-relieving drugs.

Every unnatural drug has side effects. It cannot be otherwise. It is simply what happens when you block biochemical pathways. Some of these side effects create new diseases that have been termed "iatrogenic", which means "physician caused". Some statistics suggest that iatrogenic diseases are now our nation's third leading cause of death, after heart disease and cancer.

Death is the most permanent side effect of all. In Canada, MP Terence Young issued a report suggesting that 20,000 Canadians may be killed each year from prescription drugs that are properly prescribed and properly administered. If this same ratio applies to the U.S., then 180,000 Americans may be killed each year by their pharmaceuticals.

Natural health practitioners often fall into the trap of treating the labelled condition rather than its cause(s). They look for a specific remedy for each abnormal bodily state, and often there are many from which to choose. Textbook answers tend to be oversimplified, focusing on only one aspect of a particular health challenge. So do research studies, especially those funded by companies seeking to promote their products. Both of these resources completely ignore biochemical individuality, the overriding consideration when it comes to causality.

The upside of using natural remedies to treat symptoms is that no harm is ever done. Vitamins and food-based medicines have never killed anyone. Unless the remedy corrects the cause(s) of the problem for the particular individual, however, there are two potential downsides: (1) false hope, and (2) lifelong dependence on the remedy for symptomatic relief.

Cardiovascular disease is our number one killer. There are many natural products on the market for this condition, most of which are promoted as being all one ever needs to prevent or reverse the problem. If only it were that simple. With one notable exception, all of these products treat only the symptoms. Herbal heart drops act as a heart tonic and circulatory stimulant. L-carnitine can supplement the body's own internal production of this antioxidant. Similarly, coenzyme Q_{10} can supplement the body's own production of this antioxidant. Vitamin C and lysine together strengthen the collagen in artery walls. Vitamin E is an antioxidant that also keeps platelets from sticking together, thus improving the flow characteristics of the blood. Garlic tends to normalize blood pressure. Selenium is an antioxidant that also reduces inflammation and helps to normalize blood pressure. None of these products, however, whether taken by itself or in combination with any or all of the others, is capable of removing the atherosclerotic plaque which is the ultimate cause of cardiovascular disease. There is only one complex formula that has been time proven to be able to do just that – as explained in the chapter, "Unplug the Arteries".

LAYERS OF CAUSES

Most health conditions are multifactorial in nature, meaning that there are a number of contributing factors. For arthritis, as an example, those factors could include hereditary predisposition, allergies, nutrient deficiencies, adrenal weakness, and/or stress. Never take the label of any condition as meaning anything in particular. Play a detective game to see what cause-and-effect relationships you can discover on your own. The typical advice given for any particular condition may be intended to resolve an issue that has little or nothing to do with how this condition came about in your unique body.

To simplify your detective work, I have organized parts of this book into chapters that focus on underlying themes, or deeper causes. These themes include: **digestive weaknesses** (43 symptoms), **food allergies** (187 symptoms), **toxicity** (22 symptoms), **nutrient deficiencies** (50 symptoms), **hypoglycemia** (16 symptoms), **low thyroid** (34 symptoms), **adrenal weakness** (19 symptoms), **free radical damage** (7 symptoms), **candidiasis** (23 symptoms), and **leaky gut** (17 symptoms).

Ten fundamental weaknesses can collectively trigger over 400 symptoms, some of which overlap (i.e., the same symptom can have multiple causes). The chances are excellent that whatever chronic symptoms you have are either caused or aggravated by one or more of these 10 causative themes. Supporting your particular weakness(es), may enable you to eliminate your entire cluster of symptoms, whether or not they have been given a disease name – and also to correct minor problems before they develop into major health challenges. It is by concentrating on fundamental causes that I have been able to present throughout this book 22 nutritional therapies that can be of benefit to some 88 conditions.

MENTAL INFLUENCES

Thoughts are powerful. The things we say to ourselves in our head every day (especially beliefs and judgments) have a profound influence on which diseases we attract. It is as if the body dutifully and symbolically acts out the subliminal messages we continually give it.

Someone who believes that she does not have the right to express negative feelings increases her susceptibility to cancer. Carrying secret griefs, resentments, or hatreds eats away at one psychologically – just as the disease eats away at one physically. If you know someone who has died of cancer, you will know what I am about to say is true. The personalities of cancer victims can vary from indrawn and stoical to outgoing and exuberant; but the one thing they all have in common is that you never know what is really bothering them. They may have a "what's the use" or "can't fight city hall" or "why complain when no one listens" attitude – or they may be always looking on the bright side or using the power of positive thinking, all the while denying the issues that are destroying them inside.

A friend of mine who was a visionary nutrition educator came down with breast cancer. When I explained that (a) breast problems symbolically represent refusing to nourish oneself by putting others first, and (b) cancer can be caused by refusing to express negative feelings, she immediately grasped both concepts and blurted out, "My husband, John, is such a nice guy, who could get mad at him?" Bullseye. She both put her husband first and also denied her negative feelings toward him. If she had been able to express her painful feelings, perhaps she would have been able to overcome her cancer.

Someone who resists love increases his vulnerability to heart attacks. Such people tend to be hard-driving "type A" personalities who are task oriented and achievement motivated. If your father died of a heart attack, you will know what I mean. You probably knew he loved you by what he did for you; but did ever actually say that he loved you?

There are proportionately more heart disease survivors than there are cancer survivors. This is because it is easier for the hard driving task oriented individual to switch his focus to making heart health his achievement – than it is for the cancer stricken person even to believe that a cure is possible. Someone who does not feel entitled to express negative feelings tends to be unreceptive to help because it is so unfamiliar. If you don't tell others what is wrong, then they don't know that you are in trouble and are unable to help, making you feel that your whole life is hopeless. Cancer survivors have to take a huge emotional leap that heart disease survivors do not.

Every disorder involves a mental component, to some degree or other. Back problems may symbolize not feeling supported by life. Hip problems may symbolize fear of moving forward in major decisions. Adrenal weakness relates to feeling overwhelmed and defeated – low thyroid to not feeling that you have a life of your own – a sore throat to holding back angry words – a stiff neck to not feelings safe to see other viewpoints – and on, and on, and on. The more serious the health problem, the deeper are the thoughts and feelings that are being resisted.

How to release the mental/emotional blocks that contribute to disease is the subject of another book. For this one, it is important simply to be aware of the extent to which a person's beliefs can either facilitate healing or interfere with it.

A young woman came to me excitedly exclaiming, "I am so happy to be here. I have been waiting three weeks to get this appointment, and I just know that it is going to work!" With that enthusiasm, how could it not?

Satisfied clients would often refer their husband, mother, or sister to see me. Those who came out of a sense of obligation or to humor their loved one (rather than from genuine desire) rarely followed through with my suggestions, or if they did it was only half-heartedly. They either didn't want to be helped or didn't believe that I could help them, and they acted in a way that confirmed their wish or their belief.

IT BEGINS WITH DIGESTION

Digestion is an intimate, transformative process. We take in raw materials from the outside world and transform them into the substances our bodies need to survive and thrive. What once had life in plants and animals finds new life in our bodies.

Cultures that forage and hunt for their food are very close to this transformative process. On a daily basis they take the lives of plants and animals in order that their own lives may continue. Such peoples often consider the act of eating to be very special, even sacred. They tend to see eating as part of a natural cycle, knowing that when they die their bodies will become food for worms, plants or even wild animals.

Food foragers benefit from their proximity to nature in two very interesting ways: (1) the food they eat is whole and natural, undergoing very little change from the time it was alive until the time it is consumed, and (2) the respect with which they view eating itself fosters a harmonious inner state that facilitates the process of digestion.

People in industrialized societies have mostly forgotten their connection to and dependence upon nature. Much of their food is the product of technology and bears little or no resemblance to anything that has ever lived. Food that lacks life cannot sustain life.

The western approach to eating also interferes with digestion. Food eaten quickly or in an unsettled mental state may contribute more to toxicity than to health. We have much to learn from those who live their lives simply and close to nature.

Digestion is the first step in transforming food into the living tissues of our bodies and into the fuel needed to keep those tissues functioning. It is here we need to pay particular attention. It is impossible to be in perfect health with poor digestion.

PSYCHOLOGICAL FACTORS

Every state of mind is experienced by the digestive tract. Emotions affect the flow of digestive enzymes, the emptying time of the stomach, the quality and quantity of bile, the motion of the small intestine, mucus secretions, the quality of bacteria that grow in the gut, and the elimination of wastes. Tension and strain strangle digestion. Relaxation and tranquillity allow it to flow smoothly.

The taste, smell, feel, sight and even the thought of food stimulate the secretion of saliva, the flow of gastric juice and the release of insulin. If one has no appetite, or if food does not smell or taste good, then digestive juices do not flow adequately.

The nervous and digestive systems are closely connected. Stress is an excessive form of sympathetic nervous stimulation that both impedes the movement of food through the digestive tract and inhibits the secretion of mucus needed to protect its lining. Hurried, hard-driving, critical, worrisome people tend to develop ulcers. Anxious, tense, irritable people may develop bowel problems.

When we are angry, upset or overtired, we are not able to digest our foods very well. At these times the body is preoccupied with other concerns and does not have much energy to devote to digestion. If we persist in eating at such times, we may experience indigestion and force our bodies to consume more than they are capable of handling, resulting in toxic overload. You have probably noticed that you are not really hungry when you are overstressed. Listen to your body's wisdom. Eat only when genuinely hungry – not by the clock and not for social reasons.

That stressful emotions affect digestion in a negative way is only one side of the coin. The other is that peaceful emotions affect it in a positive way. Our digestive tracts need emotional harmony almost as much as they need food.

It is beneficial to take a few minutes before each meal to create a peaceful environment within. Relax. Give silent thanks or appreciation for the meal you are about to receive. Anything you can do to clear or ease your mind will aid digestion.

HUNGER AND APPETITE

Hunger is the name given to those physiological sensations caused by the lack of food. Appetite is the psychological desire for food in order to taste and enjoy it.

Hunger usually manifests as strong, mildly painful contractions of the stomach and/or by an overwhelming desire to eat. Sometimes it may present as weakness, light-headedness, or irritability. Hunger is regulated by centres in the hypothalamus. Messages received by the hypothalamus during eating reduce hunger as food is chewed, swallowed and starts to fill the stomach. The amount by which hunger declines during eating is nature's attempt to match the amount of food taken in with what can be processed by the intestines at any given time. Hunger also strives to maintain an intake of food consistent with appropriate blood levels of key nutrients.

Appetite is quite different. It is a psychological desire for food that may exceed the body's actual need for food. A person that has satisfied hunger may still crave more. Hunger is usually for food in general. Appetite is more likely to involve certain foods that a person finds particularly enjoyable or even addictive.

Cravings for a specific food can sometimes be caused by the body's need for a particular nutrient that it provides. This phenomenon is referred to as specific hunger. Women who crave chocolate only at certain times of their menstrual cycle, for example, may do so because of its magnesium content. [*Magnesium deficiency can be a causative factor in premenstrual syndrome.*]

Cravings for a specific food are very often caused by allergy to that food. Allergy and addiction are, in effect, two sides of the same coin. Food or drink to which one is allergic gives the body an adrenalin rush, or the feeling of a "lift." As the effect wears off, the body feels tired, weak or even depressed. Each letdown triggers the desire for another lift, and hence more of the offending substance. Any food that one cannot do without on a daily basis is most likely an allergen.

DIGESTION AND WEIGHT

One contributing factor to being overweight can be sluggish digestion. Not enough food is broken down, absorbed and assimilated. Bodily cells still hunger for missing nutrients, driving the person to eat even more. "Starving to death on a full stomach" is an expression that applies to far too many people in the western world.

Anything that poor digestion causes, improved digestion can correct. By supporting digestive weaknesses, there can be an unexpected side benefit: hunger diminishes and weight is easier to control.

Sometimes people eat too much simply because they eat too quickly. By chewing slowly and taking time to experience all of the tastes and aromas of the food, one tends to enjoy meals more while eating less.

The timing of what one eats also affects one's weight. A meal eaten when one is active provides energy for immediate physical and mental activity. That same meal eaten when one is inactive, however, will cause the body to divert much of the energy provided by that meal to storage fat. For that reason, it is best to have the largest meal in the middle of the day, when one is most active. Your body would probably prefer evening meals to be light and to consume nothing after nine PM.

Obesity and overweight have many possible causes. Poor digestion is only one. Anything that can make digestion more efficient will necessarily improve health, but may not always result in losing unwanted pounds. There could be other causative factors at work, such as psychological problems, hidden food allergies, low thyroid, or specific nutrient deficiencies.

THE DIGESTIVE PROCESS

Digestion refers to the breaking down of food into particles small enough to enter cells. Absorption has to do with moving these minute food particles through the intestinal wall, so that they can be carried to every part of the body. Both digestion and absorption are performed by the digestive system.

Digestion is both mechanical and chemical. Mechanical action includes chewing by the teeth, churning of the stomach, and the wavelike motions (peristalsis) that propel food through the esophagus and intestines. All of these motions aid the chemical action provided by enzymes.

Enzymes are proteins that break down complex substances into simpler ones. They function as catalysts by speeding up chemical reactions. Digestion is highly enzyme dependent. If enzymes and digestive juices are not secreted in adequate amounts, food cannot be broken down and absorbed efficiently.

Each enzyme is specific to one kind of food molecule. Amylase hydrolyses starch into maltose, a double sugar (disaccharide). Maltase splits maltose into two molecules of glucose, a simple sugar (monosaccharide). Lipases split fats into fatty acids and glycerol. Proteases split proteins into amino acids.

The rate of movement of food through the digestive tract and the activity of digestive organs need to be controlled within optimal ranges. If food moves too slowly or too quickly, or if digestive secretions are inadequate, the body cannot be properly nourished. If digestive secretions are excessive, they may damage the lining of the gastrointestinal tract.

The body regulates its rate of digestion in two ways. The first is through nervous control. The autonomic nervous system regulates digestive activity through nerves in the sub-mucosa and muscle walls of the digestive organs. The parasympathetic part of the autonomic nervous system speeds up digestive activity, and the sympathetic part slows it down.

The second method of controlling the rate of digestion is by secretion of hormones. At various stages in the digestive process, hormones are secreted into the blood that travel to and affect other links in the digestive chain.

THE MOUTH

Digestion begins in the mouth. Teeth tear and grind down food into manageable particles and mix it with saliva, which softens and lubricates the mass. Saliva contains amylase (ptyalin), the enzyme that begins the chemical digestion of (a) plant starches (amylose and amylopectin) by converting them to dextrins, maltose, and isomaltose, and (b) animal starch (glycogen) by initiating its breakdown into glucose. [*Optimum pH for ptyalin activity is 6.9*].

Saliva also reduces bacterial growth and helps to keep the teeth and mouth clean. Its amylase enzyme breaks down the starch particles that stick between teeth after eating.

The tinier the particles that food is chewed into, the more easily it can be attacked by ptyalin in the mouth and other enzymes further down the digestive tract. Chewing food into a paste before swallowing is the most efficient way to optimize this process.

Washing down food with fluids dilutes the effect of ptyalin. Better to sip water or other beverages when the mouth is completely empty, between mouthfuls or at the end of a meal.

THE STOMACH

After leaving the mouth, a bolus of food is propelled down the esophagus by peristalsis, through the diaphragm and into the stomach. It enters via the lower esophageal sphincter (also called the cardiac sphincter).

When food reaches the stomach, the mucosa of the lower stomach and duodenum release the hormone, gastrin, into the venous blood. From there gastrin flows into the liver and the general circulation. When it reaches the stomach, gastrin stimulates gastric acid secretion and also causes the lower esophageal sphincter and ileocecal sphincter to relax. It also has a mild effect on the motility of the small intestine and gallbladder.

The introduction of protein and fat into the stomach stimulates the secretion of cholecystokinin (CCK) into the blood. This hormone slows the rate of stomach emptying and prepares for the final digestion of most foods in the small intestine.

Stimulated by gastrin, special cells in the stomach lining secrete gastric juice containing hydrochloric acid (about 0.2 percent to 0.5 percent), pepsinogen, gastric lipase and intrinsic factor (a substance that facilitates the absorption of vitamin B_{12}). Other cells secrete mucus to protect the stomach lining from being eaten away by this strong acid. A proper balance of mucus is necessary. Too much impairs digestion by reducing the concentration of acid and enzymes. Too little allows the acid to corrode the walls of the stomach.

Pepsinogen is an inactive enzyme. Hydrochloric acid (HCl) converts this enzyme into pepsin, its active form. Pepsin breaks down proteins into proteoses, peptones and polypeptides.

The main functions of hydrochloric acid are to activate pepsin and to provide the acid medium favorable for pepsin's activity (ideally pH 1.5 to 2). It is the pepsin rather than the HCl that actually breaks down proteins. Almost every type of protein in the diet is first acted upon by this enzyme.

Hydrochloric acid also liquefies the food, softens the connective tissue (collagen) in meat, hydrolyses sucrose, and precipitates casein from liquid milk protein.

As the stomach churns it mixes food, gastric juice and mucus together to form the semi-liquid substance, chyme. During this process a number of things happen, including: (1) pepsinogen is converted into pepsin, (2) proteins are converted to proteoses, peptones and polypeptides, (3) emulsified fats (triglycerides) are broken into fatty acids and glycerol, (4) inorganic minerals are ionized, and (5) the acid environment halts the digestion of starches temporarily.

The stomach also secretes water, large amounts of which are required for digestion – to produce digestive juices, to dilute food to move it more easily through the digestive tract, and to provide the medium for the chemical action of enzymes. Because water is added to food molecules as they are split by enzymes, this process is sometimes referred to as hydrolysis.

Although the whole of the stomach's contents are squeezed and churned, there is a layering effect. What one eats first tends to be kept somewhat separate from what is eaten later in the same meal. Large lumps of poorly chewed food are held longer in the stomach. If they reach the pyloric valve too soon, they are squirted back for further digestion. Fluids drunk while there is food is in the stomach pass around the solid mass and into the duodenum.

A well-chewed meal of mixed solids tends to stay in a well-functioning stomach for anywhere from one to five hours. (Insufficient chewing or overeating, however, can delay these times.) Light liquids normally leave the stomach within minutes of entering. Fruit may take 20 to 30 minutes to leave the stomach (and may be completely digested within one to two hours from the time they were eaten.) Vegetables stay in the stomach a little longer than fruits (and a lot longer if they are served with oils or sauces). Grains and starchy foods take more time than vegetables. Grain/legume combinations take longer still. Protein foods require considerable time in the stomach. Of all the solids, however, fats pass through the stomach most slowly and delay its emptying more than any other kind of food.

Spices, coffee and tea are stimulants. They increase churning of the stomach and may accelerate the emptying of its contents. If taken in excess, they can irritate the stomach walls. Excesses of salt and alcohol have the potential to destroy stomach cells.

THE SMALL INTESTINE

When the stomach has done all that it can, the pyloric sphincter at its base opens to let the chyme enter the duodenum, the first part of the small intestine. Glands in the duodenal wall secrete mucus to protect the small intestine from the strongly acidic chyme.

Acidified food entering the duodenum stimulates the pancreas to secrete a neutralizing alkaline fluid containing digestive enzymes. The stronger the acidity of the food entering the duodenum, the more of this pancreatic juice is released. The acid stimulates the mucosa of the duodenum to release more cholecystokinin (CCK) into the blood. This hormone (a) causes the gallbladder to contract and release bile, (b) stimulates the release of pancreatic enzymes and pancreatic fluid, and (c) promotes the secretion of insulin into the blood. (Insulin regulates the synthesis of pancreatic amylase.)

Pancreatic fluid and bile enter the duodenum either through a common duct, or through two ducts that are very close together, depending on anatomical differences among individuals. Pancreatic juice is mildly alkaline. It contains sodium bicarbonate plus a mixture of enzymes (pancreatin), which functions best in an alkaline medium. The enzymes in pancreatin include: (1) three proteases (chymotrypsinogen, trypsinogen, peptidase) to digest proteins, (2) a lipase (steapsin) which splits fats into monoglycerides, fatty acids and glycerol, (3) an amylase that continues the hydrolysation of starches, dextrins and glycogen that was begun by salivary amylase, (4) nucleinase, which converts nucleic acids into nucleotides, and (5) nucleotidase, which converts nucleotides into nucleosides and phosphoric acid.

Two of the pancreatic protease enzymes are first produced in inactive forms, then activated by other enzymes once they reach the small intestine. Chymotrypsinogen becomes activated into chymotrypsin, which splits proteins into proteoses, peptones and polypeptides. Trypsinogen becomes activated into trypsin, which splits specific links in the peptide chain. Peptidase, already produced in active form, comes into play only when proteins are broken down into polypeptides. These it hydrolyses into individual amino acids and small peptides (dipeptides and tripeptides).

The gallbladder stores and concentrates bile up to four times the strength it was when produced in the liver. Bile contains bile salts, cholesterol, lecithin, pigments, mucin, plus other organic and inorganic substances. Bile alkalinizes the acidic chyme so that digestion can continue in the small intestine.

Bile salts emulsify fats. They break up fats into tiny droplets that can be acted upon more efficiently by pancreatic lipase. This emulsification increases the surface area of fats by 10,000-fold. If there is an insufficiency of either bile or lipase, fats either (a) are expelled with the feces in undigested form, or (b) combine with minerals to form insoluble soaps in the colon, thereby contributing to constipation. The emulsifying action of bile aids in the absorption of fat and fat soluble vitamins from the small intestine. Bile also acts as a laxative or purgative by stimulating peristalsis of the small and large intestines.

From the duodenum, food substances descend into the next section of the small intestine, the jejunum – and from there into its final section, the ileum. It is in the 6 metres or so of the small intestine that most digestion and absorption takes place. Virtually all nutrients are absorbed through the intestinal walls. Only alcohol is absorbed through the stomach wall.

Most chemical changes that happen in the small intestine are the result of the pancreatic enzymes. Enterocrinin, a hormone, adds to this action by simulating the flow of intestinal juice. This juice contains a number of additional enzymes: (1) peptidases that convert polypeptides into single amino acids, dipeptides and tripeptides, (2) disaccharidases that split double sugars (disaccharides) into simple sugars (monosaccharides), (3) intestinal lipase that further splits fats, (4) phosphatases that separate out absorbable phosphorus from certain compounds, (5) nucleinase that converts nucleic acid into nucleotides, and (6) nucleotidase that splits nucleotides into nucleosides and phosphoric acid.

Final digestion of carbohydrates occurs mainly at the mucosal lining of the upper jejunum, and declines as they proceed down the small intestine. Disaccharidase enzymes (lactase, sucrase, maltase, isomaltase) produced by intestinal mucosal cells break down disaccharides. Lactase breaks down lactose (milk sugar) into glucose and galactose. Sucrase (also called invertase) breaks down sucrose (table sugar) into fructose (levulose) and glucose (dextrose). Maltase and isomaltase hydrolyse maltose and isomaltose, respectively, into glucose (dextrose). [_Note_: _sugars (disaccharides) are digested only in the small intestine._]

The inner surface of the small intestine outcrops into millions of tiny, finger-like filaments called villi. Each villus in turn is covered with its own microscopic projections called microvilli (also referred to as a brush border). These projections increase the absorptive surface of the intestinal lining some 600 times. They also act as a filter to prevent undesirable materials from entering the bloodstream while allowing nutrients to pass through. The microvilli also contain the disaccharidase enzymes and transporter proteins to assist in absorption. The process of absorption is highly dependent on the condition of this intricate and delicate intestinal lining.

At the base of the villi are crypts, where new epithelial cells are formed and then migrate upward to the villi. Certain cells in the crypts produce mucus for lubricating the gastrointestinal tract. Others are the source of some digestive juices. Also located in the crypts are glandular cells that signal the initiation and coordination of digestive processes.

Throughout the small intestine, enzymes continue to work on food material. Proteins are eventually broken down into single amino acids, dipeptides and tripeptides. Carbohydrates become simple sugars (glucose, fructose, galactose). Fats are split into fatty acids and glycerol (glycerine). Simple sugars and amino acids (including some dipeptides and tripeptides) are absorbed directly into the bloodstream through capillary walls in the villi. From here they pass through the portal system to the liver, where they are stored, modified or released as needed. Glucose (dextrose) is readily available to the tissues as soon as it enters the bloodstream. Fructose and galactose, however, are converted into glucose by the liver before they can be released into general circulation.

Fats do not pass directly into the bloodstream. Instead, they enter the lymphatic system via vessels called lacteals. (Lacteal means "like milk" and is so named because fat droplets in lymph fluid give it a milky appearance.) The mixture of lymph and fat that leave the small intestine is called chyle. It circulates in the lymph and enters the bloodstream via the thoracic duct (near the heart) only as the general circulation is ready and able to accept it, thus preventing the blood from becoming overloaded with fats.

Vitamins and minerals are also absorbed from the small intestine. Minerals and the water-soluble vitamins (C, B-complex) are absorbed directly into the blood. Fat soluble vitamins (A, D, E) are incorporated into fats and absorbed with them into the lymph.

Minerals are absorbed through the intestinal wall in a unique way. Stomach acid breaks down mineral compounds in food into electromagnetically charged ions (e.g., potassium chloride or KCl separates into K^+ and Cl^-.) Amino acids (from protein digestion) surround the mineral ions, neutralizing their electromagnetic charge, in a process known as "chelation". If this didn't happen, positively charged mineral ions would stick to the intestinal wall (which has a slight negative charge) and negatively charged ions would be repelled by it. For efficient mineral absorption, then, two conditions are necessary: (1) There must be sufficient hydrochloric acid in the stomach, both to separate mineral compounds into their ionic forms and to initiate the breakdown of proteins into amino acids, and (2) there must be enough protein eaten at the same time to provide sufficient amino acids for this purpose. Thus, it is best to take mineral supplements on a full stomach, when both HCl and protein are in abundant supply.

Intestinal absorption is site-specific. Minerals are absorbed in the duodenum. Protein, water-soluble vitamins and carbohydrates are absorbed in the jejunum. The ileum absorbs fat, fat-soluble vitamins, cholesterol and bile salts.

THE LIVER

In addition to producing bile from cholesterol, the liver is more importantly the chemical factory of the body. Most of the nutrients absorbed through the intestinal walls are taken by the portal circulation directly to the liver for storage, repackaging, or combining with other compounds before they can be distributed to the various cells of the body. Waste products and other potentially toxic substances either produced in the body or absorbed from the intestine are detoxified in the liver. Many compounds essential to growth and repair of bodily tissues are manufactured and/or stored in the liver. These include proteins, fats, glucose, cholesterol and lipoproteins. Since everything coming from the intestines must be processed by the liver, this organ can become overloaded. Overwork interferes with its functioning.

The liver takes simple sugars from the blood and converts them to glycogen, a storage molecule that resembles a starch. In this capacity it prevents the general circulation from being deluged with sugar (glucose). The liver also takes amino acids that have been absorbed by the small intestine and reassembles them to form various proteins, as needed. It modifies fats so that they can be used more efficiently by cells throughout the body.

The liver is the primary storehouse for vitamins A, D, E, K, B_{12}, C, copper, iron, and glycogen. The liver also regulates blood levels of such substances as glucose and vitamin A, and releases them as needed to maintain constant concentrations in the blood. It also converts some vitamins to their biologically active form (e.g., beta-carotene to retinol, vitamin B_6 to pyridoxal phosphate).

LARGE INTESTINE

Humans do not have the enzymes needed to digest all of the complex carbohydrates (polysaccharides) that they consume. The cell walls of plants are indigestible and constitute what is commonly referred to as "dietary fiber" (consisting of celluloses, hemicelluloses, pectins and lignin). Fiber is critical to the healthy functioning of the large intestine (or colon), a convoluted tube that only empties when full. Fiber comes only from unrefined plant foods and not from foods of animal origin (e.g., meat, fish, poultry, eggs, dairy products). Fiber fills out the colon, softens the stool, lessens the pressure on the colonic wall, and eases excretion of the stool.

After the small intestine has absorbed all that it can, fiber and non-digestible waste material pass from the ileum into the large intestine. The ileocecal valve prevents waste from travelling backward into the small intestine. Large quantities of mucus (but no enzymes) are secreted by the large intestine. Bacteria that are normal inhabitants of the large intestine degrade some previously undigested materials and act on food residues to produce vitamin K and biotin, only a tiny amount which is absorbed through the colon wall.

In the colon, water mixes with the fecal mass to bring it to the right consistency to pass easily from the body. Excess water used in the digestive process is reabsorbed back into the body, to prevent dehydration.

Many strains of microbes exist in the large intestine; however, *Lactobacillus*, *Streptococcus* and *Diplococcus* are among the most common. Proportions of intestinal flora vary according to the kinds of food consumed. A diet high in complex carbohydrates promotes beneficial gram-positive fermentative flora, while a low fiber diet increases potentially harmful gram-negative putrefactive bacteria.

At intervals, when the colon is full, involuntary muscles within its wall propel solid waste material (feces) toward the rectum. During defecation, these feces (or stools) are eliminated from the body by both involuntary and voluntary muscle actions. Fecal material contains bacteria, undigested plant fiber, intestinal secretions, and cellular debris from the gastrointestinal tract. In those on a typical western diet, the bulk of the feces consists of bacteria. Bile salts in the stools give them their characteristic yellowish-brown color.

Bile acts as a natural laxative that promotes healthy colon function. Without adequate bile, large blobs of fats pass through the gut undigested and combine with minerals to form insoluble soaps - leading to constipation, poor mineral absorption, and osteoporosis.

Bowel transit time is very important to health. Delayed emptying encourages putrefaction and bile acids to combine to form free radicals in the colon (e.g., apcholic acid, 3-methyl cholanthrene). These renegade molecules not only damage the colon but are also absorbed into the body where they become causative factors for atherosclerosis and cancer.

Dietary fiber is paramount for healthy colon function. In addition, a sufficient daily water intake (e.g., two litres) and regular exercise (such as walking) also help to promote healthy elimination. A well-functioning colon will deliver from one to three bowel movements per day, from food that was consumed in the last 24 hours. Rarely is this ideal achieved in practise, at least not on the typical western diet.

INTESTINAL IMMUNITY

The secretions that pour into the digestive tract not only digest food but also protect against foreign invaders. One of the functions of hydrochloric acid, for example, is to destroy foreign organisms and inhibit the multiplication of pathogenic bacteria. The bactericidal and bacteriostatic actions of HCl provide protection against some forms of food poisoning and help to control intestinal flora. Insufficient stomach acid may fail to sterilize food enough to prevent undesirable bacteria from growing in the digestive tract.

A stomach that produces sufficient acidity and proteolytic enzymes can break down potentially antigenic (allergy-causing) proteins and viruses before they cause harm. Protease enzymes from the pancreas also help to keep the small intestine free from parasites. Saliva and intestinal mucus contain immunoglobulin A, which can bind bacterial toxins and inactivate certain parasites. Bile is an antiseptic that helps to keep the small intestine free of disease-causing microbes.

A small percentage of bacteria ingested with food do survive the acidic environment of the stomach and the alkaline action of the bile to reach the lower intestine and colon, where they thrive and play a symbiotic role in our health.

RECYCLING AND RENEWAL

Most enzymes and fluids secreted in the gastrointestinal tract are reabsorbed. Enzymes and mucus are broken down and digested along with dietary proteins. Bile is largely recycled. Most fluid is reabsorbed in the small intestine; however, final absorption of excess water and electrolytes occurs in the colon.

Cells that line the gastrointestinal tract continually die and are replaced with new ones. Those in the intestinal villi turn over rapidly, sometimes within two or three days. The lifespan of colonic cells can be as little as from three to eight days. That means that a diseased intestine can potentially renew itself within days – provided that all sources of the original problem are eliminated and the condition was not too far advanced.

Some of the epithelial cells that are sloughed off high enough in the gastrointestinal tract may be broken down into amino acids and absorbed through the intestinal wall. The rest are excreted in the feces.

DIGESTIVE SUMMARY

Breakdown of carbohydrates begins in the mouth with salivary amylase, which begins the hydrolysis of starches. From there, very little happens to complex carbohydrates until they reach the upper small intestine, where most carbohydrate digestion continues. Here, pancreatic amylase reduces complex carbohydrates to disaccharides. Enzymes in the microvilli split these disaccharides into simple sugars (monosaccharides), which are then absorbed through the intestinal mucosa into the bloodstream.

Digestion of protein begins in the stomach with acid denaturation and pepsin attack, then continues in the small intestine with pancreatic trypsin, chymotrypsin and other proteases. In the process, proteins are fully degraded to free amino acids and small peptides, then absorbed through the intestinal wall into the bloodstream.

Breakdown of emulsified fats begins in the stomach. Breakdown of non-emulsified fats begins in the duodenum, where bile salts and lipases act on them, breaking them down into fatty acids and glycerol. This breakdown continues throughout the small intestine. Most fatty acids are absorbed through the intestinal wall into the lymphatic system.

INFANTS' DIGESTION

In infancy the stomach produces rennin, an enzyme that breaks down casein (a milk protein) into paracasein. As the child matures, the ability to produce this enzyme is gradually lost. In both childhood and adult life, however, the stomach continues to produces gastric lipase, an enzyme that breaks down pre-emulsified fats (such as butter) into fatty acids and glycerol.

Infants do not produce amylase (starch-splitting) enzymes at birth and are unable to do so for quite some time. Salivary amylase (ptyalin) is not normally present in any appreciable quantity until about six months of age. Pancreatic amylase is not produced in adequate amounts until the molar teeth are fully developed – which may not be until ages of from 28 to 36 months. For these reasons, cereals, breads, crackers and other starchy foods should not be given to young infants. Unfortunately, cereal is usually the first food recommended by pediatricians and dietitians.

Infants are, however, readily able to digest proteins and fats from birth. Unlike adults, their saliva produces fat-splitting enzymes. Their stomachs produce hydrochloric acid, pepsin and fat-digesting enzymes. Their pancreases produce trypsin and steapsin. Nature obviously intends young humans to live primarily on proteins and fats for the first two years or so.

Mothers in primitive societies are more in tune with their babies' digestive needs than we are. They frequently nurse their infants for 12, 24 and even up to 36 months. The first solid food they give is usually liver or other organ meats, which mother first chews thoroughly in her own mouth and then passes to baby.

Human milk is the ideal food for babies. Cow's milk provides what calves need; humans have different requirements. Human milk has one third of the protein, one third of the minerals, and about 60 percent more carbohydrate (lactose) than found in cow's milk. The total fat content of human milk is only slightly higher than that in cow's milk but provides significantly higher amounts of essential fatty acids.

The amount of lactose (milk sugar) in human milk is higher than in any other species. It is needed for the much greater brain development that human beings have over animals. The larger proportion of protein and minerals in cow's milk, on the other hand, is needed for the very much larger body of that animal.

The lactose in human milk differs in both quantity and quality from that in cow's milk. The beta-lactose in human milk is capable of producing pure bacillus bifida flora in the infant's intestinal tract. The alpha-lactose in cow's milk cannot.

In the small intestine, lactose is broken down into two simple sugars, galactose and glucose (dextrose). Galactose is the only source material that develops the myelin sheath, the coating that surrounds all nerves. Lactose is the only source of galactose. Feeding infants any other sugar (e.g., sucrose, dextrose, maltose, honey, corn syrup, molasses) may delay or impair the myelination of their nervous tissues and brain.

The protein in human milk is about 60 percent whey and 40 percent casein. Cow's milk is 85 percent casein and only 15 percent whey. Whey proteins are water soluble; casein is not. The fact that mother's milk has four times more whey than cow's milk makes it very easy to digest. Infants can use 100 percent of the protein in breast milk, but only 50 percent in cow's milk. Of the remaining 50 percent, some is not digested but excreted in the feces, and some is absorbed into the bloodstream but not utilized. Thus it causes extra stress on little kidneys. In order to get enough protein, the bottle-fed baby must ingest more milk than the breast-fed child. In so doing he must take in a larger total volume of food, thus contributing to possible overweight.

The amino acid profile of human and cow's milk are also quite different. Between three and four times as much cow's milk protein must be ingested to provide the same quantity of cysteine (an amino acid) as that provided by human milk.

The fat in human milk is about eight percent linoleic acid. Cow's milk fat provides only three percent of this essential fatty acid. Breast milk also contains dihommogamma-linolenic acid (DGLA), which is absent in cow's milk and most other human foods. DGLA is an intermediate in the production of PG1 prostaglandins, which have beneficial effects on immune system function, kidney function, blood pressure and clotting ability. Unheated breast milk also contains fat-splitting enzymes that are absent in pasteurized milks from any source.

Human milk has about 10 times more vitamin E than cow's milk, twice as much vitamin A, and less than half as much of vitamins B$_2$ and B$_6$. Cow's milk has about seven times as much phosphorus and five times as much sodium as human milk.

Breast milk also protects infants from infections. It is the means by which mother transfers to baby's body such anti-infective substances as immunoglobulins, lactoferrin, leucocytes and complement.

Feeding infants inappropriate foods may not provide them with enough of the nutrients they require for proper growth and development. It also may contribute to toxicity by overloading their tiny systems with indigestible factors and excesses of nutrients they do not need. Furthermore, it may contribute to the development of allergies. The two most common classes of food that westerners give their babies before their digestive systems can handle them are cereal grains (especially wheat) and cow's milk. Allergies to wheat and dairy products are two of the most common allergies affecting adults. What we feed our children now can affect them for life.

INTESTINAL FLORA

In our intestines live thriving communities of microorganisms. We give them a warm place to live and food to eat. In return, they (a) provide us with important immune protection, (b) help us with digestion and elimination, and (c) supply a sprinkling of vitamins (K, B-12, pantothenic acid, pyridoxine, and biotin). Most of these vitamins are produced too low in the gut to be absorbed, however. Perhaps our internal ecosystem extends beyond our bodies. Maybe it was nature's design that our vitamin-fortified feces might enrich the soil to which they are returned, for the benefit of the micro-inhabitants that live there.

A properly functioning stomach has enough acidity to prevent indigenous microflora from growing there. During periods of very low acidity, however, some microbes can manage to pass through to the stomach from the intestines.

If the liver and gallbladder are functioning well, very few microorganisms can live in the duodenum. That is because bile inhibits their growth. The lower small intestine, however, teams with colonies of *Staphylococcus, Lactobacillus, Streptobacillus, Veillonella,* and *Clostridium perfringens.*

The large intestine has an even greater abundance of tiny inhabitants. They include (a) gram-positive *Clostridium* species, (b) gram-negative *Bacteroides* and *Fusobacterium* species, (c) anaerobes such as *Escherichia coli, Enterobacter aerogenes, Proteus, Pseudomonas, Enterococcus, Lactobacillus,* and *Mycoplasma.*

The colon is also host to many fungi, protozoa and viruses. Such microflora are opportunists. They do not cause disease until the balance among competing microorganisms is upset, or until they lodge in other parts of the body.

The presence of microbes in the gut is a constant stimulus to the immune system. They give it lots of practise in making antibodies to foreign invaders, thus enhancing protection against disease-causing agents. By simply taking up space in the gut and eating the nutrients there, our resident microflora may prevent pathogenic organisms from gaining a foothold and causing infections. Also, some resident microbes actually produce antibiotics to help eliminate invaders.

The pattern of bacterial strains in the gut is quite different from person to person and is influenced by diet. In general, those who consume high fiber, vegetarian or low meat diets tend to have more stable colonies of bacteria than those who consume diets high in meat and processed foods.

Balance among our intestinal inhabitants is important to day-to-day health. It is the normal state in which the beneficial microbes keep the potentially harmful ones in check. This delicate balance, however, can be easily upset by antibiotics, birth control pills, and steroid drugs. When this happens, certain microorganisms may flourish out of control. The most notable of these is *Candida albicans,* an opportunistic yeast that normally lives harmlessly in the eyes, mouth, intestines, urogenital tract, and on the skin. When the number of indigenous bacteria is reduced, *Candida* flourishes to cause infections of the mouth (thrush), skin and vagina and may even enter the bloodstream and respiratory tract to cause systemic candidiasis

Lactic bacteria can help both to maintain microbial balance in the gut and re-establish it once it has been lost. These special bacteria transform sugars into lactic acid. They are abundant in nature and very useful.

Lactic bacteria are necessary to the production of fermented milk (e.g., yogurt, kefir, cultured buttermilk), in the making of cheeses, in the fermentation of certain foods (e.g., sauerkraut, pickles, olives), and in the preservation of silage for animal feedings. They are also essential for the survival of both humans and animals. As normal inhabitants of the digestive system, skin and vagina they help protect those tissues against the action of harmful microbes.

Of the 400 pecies (of 40 genera) of microflora living in the human intestinal tract, nine are different strains of *Lactobacillus*. Some of these strains are found throughout the entire digestive tract, even in the highly acid stomach and in the mouth. *Lactobacilli* produce lactic acid by fermenting carbohydrates. They themselves both resist acids and survive in the alkaline bile.

Lactic acid improves digestion by enhancing intestinal peristalsis and hindering the proliferation of harmful microorganisms. Also, it tends to improve the solubility of mineral salts, thereby providing a favorable environment for the utilization and assimilation of calcium.

Lactobacillus acidophilus is the most important and most stable strain of *Lactobacilli* in the intestine. It shares the same environment with and has the ability to displace potentially harmful bacteria. It does so by producing substances that inhibit or antagonize these other bacteria. (The antibacterial substances produced by *L. acidophilus* include lactic and acetic acids, hydrogen peroxide and bacteriocins.)

At least 26 kinds of bacteria are inhibited by *L. acidophilus*, including *E. coli, Salmonella, Staphylococcus,* and *Streptococcus.* Evidence suggests that *L. acidophilus* may also improve immune response to infection by increasing the activity of macrophages and lymphocytes. Thus, *L. acidophilus* has a critical role to play in helping to protect against infection and to maintain health. Many travellers, for example, have learned that *L. acidophilus* can prevent and/or reduce diarrhea brought on by changes in drinking water.

L. acidophilus is used successfully to inhibit infections of the oral herpes simplex virus and the fungus, *Candida albicans.* Taken in a douche, it can help counteract vaginal infections, candidiasis, and urinary tract infections. Evidence also shows that, taken orally, *L. acidophilus* can have a positive effect as part of the treatment of such diverse conditions as canker sores, constipation, diarrhea, infections, irritable bowel syndrome, and ulcerative colitis.

An important benefit of *L. acidophilus* is its ability to correct antibiotic-induced imbalances in intestinal flora. Antibiotics kill harmful bacteria, but the popular broad-spectrum ones also kill the beneficial flora in our guts – the ones that are our natural defences against pathogenic bacteria, molds and fungi. Antibiotics reduce immediate infections, but at the expense of making us more vulnerable to future infections. Prolonged use of antibiotics is one of the surest way to encourage rampant growth of *Candida albicans*, which in turn provides a favorable environment for the development of allergies, chronic fatigue syndrome, and AIDS. Fortunately, we do not have to let minor imbalances become major problems. It is a simple matter to follow antibiotic treatments with supplements of *L. acidophilus*.

L. acidophilus is found in yogurt and other fermented dairy products. In these cultured foods, the *L. acidophilus* feeds on and partially breaks down the lactose (milk sugar). For this reason, some people who have difficulty in digesting lactose may find that yogurt goes down with fewer side effects than, say, milk or cheeses. Those who have a total intolerance to lactose, however, will not be able to handle yogurt. Although about 70 percent of the lactose in yogurt has been broken down by bacterial action, the 30 percent that remains is still a problem for sensitive people.

If you intend to use yogurt as a means of ingesting therapeutic levels of *L. acidophilus*, there is no benefit to buying a brand that provides multiple probiotic strains. *L. bulgaricus* and a number of other strains compete with *L. acidophilus*. Also, make sure that the yogurt was cultured after it was pasteurized and not before. The heat caused by pasteurization destroys bacterial cultures and renders them useless.

The optimum range for dietary supplementation with *L. acidophilus* appears to be from one to 10 billion active cells daily. Those who are lactose intolerant are well advised to choose *L. acidophilus* supplements that are milk-free. Successful cultures can thrive on malto-dextrins, for example, instead of lactose. For maximum shelf life, *L. acidophilus* supplements need to be kept in tightly sealed containers and refrigerated. Capsules, because of their ability to seal out the air, retain their potency longer than do powders.

FOOD COMBINING

Healthy youngsters have the amazing ability to digest just about anything they eat, in almost any combination, at any time of day. When digestive juices are at peak capacity, the entire digestive system works very efficiently. If hydrochloric acid and bile are produced in abundance, for example, they can sterilize the putrefactive by-products produced by temporary overloads. At this enviable time of life, overeating or eating unwisely does not necessarily result in indigestion.

There are some genetically rare individuals who are blessed with a generous flow of digestive juices and enzymes into their advanced years. For most of us, however, our ability to produce these vital substances declines with age. The older we get, the more attention we need to pay to the combination and timing of what we eat.

Proteins and fats stay in the stomach a long time (from three to five hours). Sugars, however pass right through the stomach and are not digested until they reach the small intestine. When concentrated proteins (and/or fats) are eaten with concentrated sugars, the stomach holds onto the whole mess until it can break down as much of the protein as it can. In the meantime, sugars are held in the stomach far longer than necessary and react with other stomach contents to ferment and form putrefactive gases. Hydrochloric acid, if produced in sufficient quantity, can neutralize the putrefactive by-products so that the person has a minimum of gastric distress. Many people over 30, however, will experience burping, bloating, belching and indigestion from such combinations.

To ease this kind of burden on the digestive tract, it is wise *not* to combine concentrated proteins and/or fats (e.g., meat, fish, poultry, eggs, cheese, milk, butter) with concentrated sugars (e.g., fruits, fruit juices, sweet and sour sauces, pastries, pies, cakes, soft drinks, candy, sweet liqueurs) at the same meal. A sweet dessert after dinner is particularly challenging to digestion. Other poor combinations include orange juice with eggs, steak followed by pie, sweet and sour sauces on meats, sugary cereals with milk, fruit salad with cottage cheese, sausages with syrupy pancakes, chicken wings with sugary barbecue sauce, and baked beans sweetened with honey or molasses. Eliminating all such protein-sugar combinations is a mandatory first step in any serious program to improve digestion.

Fruits and fruit juices are most easily digested if taken as an appetizer about 30 minutes before a meal or as a separate mini-meal unto themselves. The same goes for foods made from refined sugars, which for other health reasons ought to be consumed sparingly, if at all. (Refined sugars include white sugar, brown sugar, raw sugar, fructose/levulose, glucose/dextrose, lactose, molasses, corn syrup, and agave syrup. Honey is a sugar refined by bees, but refined nevertheless.)

It is the degree of concentration of proteins/fats and sugars that creates the difficulty. Adding small, dilute amounts of one category to the other may not be a problem. For example, adding a sprinkling of raisins to oatmeal cereal, or adding a little dried fruit to a trail mix of nuts and seeds are combinations that may be well tolerated. Foods such as whole grains, nuts, seeds and vegetables are natural mixtures of starches, proteins and fats that usually combine well with concentrated proteins or fats

Some nutritional approaches insist on elaborate rules of food combining – such as not combining starches with proteins, and not combining acid fruits with sub-acid fruits, and eating melons by themselves. Such strict rules are unnecessary for the vast majority of people. Eating only one food or food category at a time can be of temporary therapeutic benefit to someone with extremely poor digestion. In the long term, however, it makes more sense to support the digestive weakness than it does to try to avoid its symptoms.

The belief that starches are easier to digest without protein is based on the information that the acid environment of the stomach halts the action of salivary amylase. Since the acidity of the stomach is triggered by the eating of protein, then omitting protein from the meal will theoretically enable salivary amylase to continue to work on starches while they are in the stomach. Starch breakdown continues in the small intestine, however, with the action of pancreatic amylase. Most people who chew their food thoroughly and who have adequate levels of pancreatic amylase will not need to separate starches and proteins. Those who do find starches easier to digest if separated from proteins may be able to overcome this limitation by supplementing with a broad spectrum digestive aid containing pancreatin.

Fruit juices and sweetened beverages are most easily digested when consumed at least 30 minutes before or three hours after a meal. Unsweetened drinks (e.g., water, mineral water, herbal teas) may be sipped with meals without any impairment of digestion – provided they are taken when the mouth is empty and not used to dilute or wash down food. Thorough chewing is needed both to mix salivary amylase with starches in order to start their digestion and to break down food particles finely enough to prepare them for enzymatic activity further down. Drinking liquids through food impairs this process.

Drinking with meals does **not** dilute stomach acid to any appreciable extent. Gastric fluid contains only about 0.2 to 0.5 percent hydrochloric acid. It would take an impossible volume of fluid to make any significant difference in this concentration. It is not the acid that does the digesting; however, it is the pepsin that the acid activates.

DIGESTIVE ORCHESTRATION

Digestion is an intricate and well-orchestrated process that has the potential to be extremely efficient. What works well in theory does not always manifest fully in practise, however. Our desire for how much and what kind of food may exceed our bodily ability to handle foods of those quantities and qualities. Our ability to digest many kinds of foods tends to decline with age. The following are explanations of the most common digestive difficulties we are likely to experience, together with suggestions for correcting them.

OVEREATING

Overwork of the digestive system is probably the most common digestive difficulty in western countries. We tend to eat too much and too frequently. We eat even when our bodies are not genuinely hungry. We often dump more food into a stomach that is still struggling with the last challenge we gave it.

Overeating does not always result in putting on extra weight. It simply means that we are exceeding our digestive system's capacity to break down all the food we eat and eliminate all of its waste products. This is a prescription for poor health. Anything that remains undigested in the intestinal tract ferments and becomes food for bacteria, which give off gas and secrete toxic by-products that may enter the bloodstream and cause diseases. Overeating also creates a backlog for the liver, the organ that works hard (a) to process all food components that are absorbed into the bloodstream, (b) to dispose of waste products of metabolism, and (c) to neutralize all potentially harmful substances in the blood, whatever their source. If the liver is kept too busy processing food, it is unable to devote enough time to its important tasks of detoxification. Cells tend to become strangled in their own waste products, preventing them from absorbing the nutrients they need and thus shortening their lifespan.

Internal toxicity contributes to many disease processes. For that reason, many natural practitioners insist that everyone who is not in perfect health, whatever his or her condition, needs to undergo some form of detoxification (e.g., fasting, colon cleansing, detoxifying herbs).

Many people of advancing years have attributed their longevity to purposeful under-eating. They have developed the habit of leaving the table before they are completely full. Experiments also suggest that animals which are slightly underfed tend to live longer than those who are fed to capacity.

Often there are psychological reasons why people overeat. Sometimes it is simply because the food tastes so good. There is also the very prevalent concern that to be underfed is to be undernourished. The irony is that most overfed people are also undernourished. With the proliferation of food supplements available today, there is no reason why anyone needs to suffer from the deficiency of any nutrient. Much of the food we eat today is so depleted of nutrients that no matter how much we eat we are still likely to be lacking in something.

Sometimes good intentions result in overfeeding, like the mother who forces her feverish child to eat, insisting that "you have to keep up your strength." During an acute fever, the body is not hungry. Giving it solid food at that time may provide more nourishment for the invading bacteria and interfere with the liver's ability to dispose of their toxic by-products. For this reason, most natural practitioners (and some orthodox ones) advocate consuming only clear fluids during the acute phase of any illness and to resume solid food only when the body is genuinely hungry for it.

There are a number of simple guidelines we can follow to prevent overeating, such as the following: Eat only when genuinely hungry and not by the clock. Stop eating before feeling stuffed. Allow at least three hours between meals and snacks.

It can also be beneficial to take regular, mini-fasts lasting from one to three days. During such times no solid food is to be consumed, only clear fluids (e.g., vegetable juices, broths, fruit juices, herbal teas). Giving the body periodic, brief vacations from solid food enables it to catch up on its detoxification or "house-cleaning," so to speak. This detoxification can be enhanced by taking colon cleansing supplements at the same time (such as finely powdered psyllium hulls or herbal-fiber blends). Vitamin-mineral supplements may be continued during these short fasts, if desired. There is no need to make an ordeal out of a mini-fast; if at any time it becomes too uncomfortable, one can simply discontinue it and return to solid food. [Note: *Insulin-dependent diabetics should **not** fast.*]

INDIGESTION

Antacid medications are big business. Huge advertising budgets are spent to convince us that indigestion is caused by too much stomach acid and that alkalinizing drugs are the solution. This approach does provide temporary relief, but it is more beneficial to corporate profits than it is to health. And it is based on a misconception.

The most frequent cause of so-called "acid indigestion" is too *little* stomach acid, *not* too much. Without enough hydrochloric acid, food cannot be digested properly. It stays in the stomach for prolonged periods, fermenting and producing increasing amounts of gas. Taking an antacid at this point alkalinizes the stomach contents, causing them to be dropped into the small intestine. There they continue to ferment, still producing gas. Nothing has happened to improve digestion. Quite the contrary. This drastic measure halts any further digestion and merely relocates the symptom, by exchanging stomach gas for intestinal gas. Digestive difficulties have actually been made worse because the flow of bile and pancreatic enzymes depends on the acidity of food leaving the stomach, which acidity has just been eliminated by the antacid.

If hydrochloric acid levels are very low, sometimes the emptying time of the stomach is delayed for so long that bile is regurgitated backward from the duodenum into the stomach. Bile is caustic and very irritating to the stomach lining. Because bile is alkaline, it causes a reflex secretion of stomach acid to neutralize it. At this point the person will likely experience a burning sensation. Taking an antacid will relieve the burn, of course; but the stomach only became acidic after the bile had been regurgitated back into it. If there had been enough hydrochloric acid when it was needed, no burning sensation would have been experienced later.

Chronic use of antacids makes an already underactive stomach even weaker. Proteins and minerals become increasingly difficult to break down and absorb. Bodily tissues can be starving for these vital substances even when consumed in abundance. Antacid drugs also encourage bacterial overgrowth in the stomach and small intestine by reducing the acidity that is their natural antagonist.

Antacids thus contribute to degenerative diseases. Fortunately, there is a better way. Indigestion is a symptom of digestive weakness. It makes more sense to strengthen that weakness than it does to try to stifle its symptoms. Taking supplementary hydrochloric acid and digestive enzymes with meals can correct most cases of indigestion by supplying the stomach with enough acid when it is needed. The only time it is not wise to take supplementary HCl is when an ulcer is actually present. If you were to take a supplement containing HCl and you had an ulcer, you would notice a burning sensation behind the tip of the breastbone, within minutes of taking such a product. If that happens, a little dolomite or baking soda will neutralize the excess acid to provide relief within a few minutes.

FLATULENCE

Belching and breaking wind are far more than social problems. They are symptoms of incomplete digestion and potentially toxic overload.

Intestinal flatulence is caused by fermentation and rancidity in the gut. This gas contains hydrogen, methane, skatoles, indoles, carbon dioxide, nitrogen and oxygen. Putrefactive by-products frim this fermentation may be absorbed from the intestinal tract into the bloodstream. Blood carrying these toxic wastes circulates throughout the body adding an extra burden to the liver and kidneys.

If you experience burping or belching, check to see if your last meal combined proteins/fats with sugars. The simple step of eliminating such combinations has enabled many people to banish stomach gas completely.

LOW STOMACH ACID

If stomach gas persists in the absence of difficult food combinations, then low stomach acid is usually the problem. In such cases it is very helpful to take supplements providing hydrochloric acid (in the form of betaine hydrochloride or glutamic acid hydrochloride), preferably in combination with digestive enzymes.

If the body's production of hydrochloric acid is low, then the entire digestive system will be weak. Each link in the digestive chain responds to the one that precedes it. If there is not enough stomach acid, not enough pepsinogen will be converted into pepsin and proteins will not be broken down properly. If the chyme leaving the stomach is not acidified enough by HCl, insufficient pancreatic juice and bile will be secreted into the duodenum. Without sufficient bile, globs of fat combine with minerals to form insoluble soaps that may cause constipation. Virtually everyone who is chronically constipated also produces insufficient hydrochloric acid.

Legumes (e.g., beans, peas, lentils) cause gas in just about everyone, including those whose digestive systems are in top form. That is because they contain two unusual starches (raffinose and stachyose) which cannot be broken down by human intestinal enzymes. These substances pass into the colon undigested, where they are acted upon by bacteria to form carbon dioxide and hydrogen.

The indigestible starches in beans can be broken down by extremely thorough cooking. The most effective way to "de-gas" beans is the following three-step process: (1) soak the dried beans in water overnight, (2) discard this water and boil them for 15 minutes, then (3) discard this water and re-boil them until they turn to mush. Adding traditional spices and seasonings may also improve their digestibility. Most of the gas-producing starches in beans can also be eliminated by sprouting. Bean sprouts are easy on the digestive system.

ULCERS

Gastric ulcers are open sores or lesions caused by the action of hydrochloric acid and pepsin attempting to digest the stomach wall. The usual symptoms include abdominal discomfort and pain 45 to 60 minutes after a meal, or during the night. The pain may be experienced as burning, gnawing, cramping or aching. Eating a meal or taking antacids usually brings immediate but only temporary relief.

Repressed emotions, worry, stress, smoking, alcohol, ASA/aspirin compounds, and non-steroidal inflammatory drugs (NSAIDs) are all linked to the development of both gastric and duodenal ulcers. Other causative factors include a low fiber diet and hidden food allergies. If food allergy is the cause, then the ulcer will persist until the offending foods are eliminated, regardless of what other therapeutic measures may be taken.

Some studies have found a bacterium, *Helicobacter pylori*, present in peptic ulcers. This invading organism is associated with inflammation of the stomach and duodenum, which subsides when the bacterium is destroyed by antibiotics. Rather than causing ulcers, however, it may be that *H. pylori* is an opportunist which takes over once normal stomach acid levels have been reduced (e.g., from prolonged use of antacid medications).

Gastric ulcers are often caused by an uncoordinated flow of stomach acid – not enough when it is needed, and too much when it is not. Low stomach acid causes indigestion. If the person takes an antacid, this medication alkalinizes the stomach contents, causing them to be released prematurely into the duodenum – where they mix with alkaline bile and alkaline pancreatic juice. This over-alkaline mass may sometimes cause a reflux of bile back into the stomach. Bile is corrosive and triggers the stomach to release excess acid to neutralize it. Thus, the rebound surge of hydrochloric acid occurs when there is no food in the stomach.

The medical treatment for ulcers is to take drugs that reduce or eliminate stomach acid secretion. These drugs, however, impair digestion and alter the function of the cells that line the gastrointestinal tract. There is also a high relapse rate as soon as such drugs are discontinued. Rather than attempting to eliminate stomach acid (a vital bodily secretion), a more effective approach is to increase the integrity of the lining of the stomach and duodenum.

A high fiber diet both speeds the healing of peptic ulcers and prevents their recurrence. This is probably because of fiber's ability to promote the secretion of mucus and to delay gastric emptying time. A high fiber diet is one that includes generous amounts of vegetables, whole grains, nuts, seeds and fruits and excludes refined sugars and flours.

Vitamin A, vitamin C, vitamin E and zinc help to maintain the integrity of the lining of the digestive tract and prevent ulcers. There are also two natural substances that can be used therapeutically to promote the healing of an ulcerated gastrointestinal lining. These are raw cabbage juice and de-glycrrhizinated licorice (DGL).

Raw cabbage juice has a long history of treating peptic ulcers. One litre of the fresh juice, taken in divided doses throughout the day, may result in total ulcer healing in about 10 days or so. Exactly how cabbage juice works is not known. Many believe that it contains a unique ingredient (loosely dubbed "vitamin U") that is a specific for ulcer healing. Some speculate that its content of glutamine may stimulate the body's production of mucin, a glycoprotein found in mucus.

De-glycrrhizinated licorice root (DGL) is another effective anti-ulcer treatment. One study demonstrated that DGL was as effective as antacids and prescription drugs in treating duodenal ulcers, but with one important difference: there were fewer relapses in those taking DGL compared to those taking the antacids and prescription drugs. Rather than inhibit the release of acid, DGL stimulates the normal defence mechanisms that prevent ulcer formation. It helps (a) to improve the quantity and quality of the protective substances that line the stomach and intestinal tract, (b) to increase the lifespan of intestinal cells, and (c) to improve blood supply to the intestinal lining. DGL also reduces the gastric bleeding caused by aspirin. The recommended usage for DGL is to take two 300 mg. capsules either between meals or 20 minutes before meals. A course of treatment may take from two to four months, depending on individual response.

If an ulcer is present, then any digestive enzyme supplements taken should **not** contain hydrochloric acid (e.g., betaine hydrochloride, glutamic acid hydrochloride). One the ulcer has healed, however, proper acidification of the stomach may help to prevent their recurrence.

REFLUX ESOPHAGITIS

There is one type of ulcer that does not respond to conventional treatments. This is the esophageal ulcer. The esophagus lacks the thick mucus lining that would protect it from strong acids. In reflux esophagitis, stomach acid splashes upward into the esophagus creating an intense form of heartburn. If it happens often enough, ulceration of esophageal tissue is the inevitable result.

In most stomachs, gravity ensures that gastric acid flows downward and not up into the esophagus. There is only one way that stomach acid can reflux upward. That is if a small portion of the upper stomach becomes trapped or pinched in the diaphragm, a condition known as hiatal hernia. Not everyone with hiatal hernia experiences reflux esophagitis, but everyone with esophageal ulcers has a hiatal hernia.

A hiatal hernia is created by an opening in the diaphragm that is slightly too large. It is a structural problem that may flare up frequently, very rarely or never. Whenever the stomach becomes pinched in the diaphragm, the only way to relieve the problem is to restore the stomach to its proper position. This can be done in a number of ways: (1) chiropractic adjustments can relieve the muscular spasms affecting the diaphragm, causing it to release its hold on the stomach, (2) drinking two glasses of water and jumping up and down uses gravity to drop the stomach back into place, (3) allowing sunlight to shine on the forehead (or a flashlight on the bridge of the nose) for about 10 minutes stimulates a pineal reflex that relaxes the spine, that in turn relaxes the diaphragm allowing it to release the stomach, and/or (4) sleeping with the head elevated (e.g., by placing four inch blocks under the bedposts at the head of the bed) will ease the problem by prevent the backing up of gastric juices, until further corrective action can be taken.

DIARRHEA

Diarrhea is the condition whereby stools are liquid and bowel movements are frequent. It can be caused by bacterial infection from food poisoning ("turista"), from disaccharidase deficiencies, or from irritation of the colon. In acute diarrhea, especially in infants, there may be danger of dehydration and loss of salts. Diarrhea lasting more than a few days should not be taken lightly. Alternating constipation and diarrhea could be symptoms of a tumor or other blockage requiring immediate medical attention.

If the small intestine lacks the enzymes to break down disaccharides (e.g., lactose, sucrose, maltose), undigested and unabsorbed sugars remain in the gut and osmotically attract large volumes of water, thus making the stools more fluid. Sometimes the lack of disaccharidase enzymes is the cause of diarrhea and sometimes it is the effect. Severe diarrhea is known to cause temporary loss of brush border enzymes. That is why those recovering from diarrhea are usually advised to avoid milk products and sugars, which only exacerbate the problem.

Colitis and spastic colon are conditions wherein the large intestine becomes so irritated that it expels its watery contents profusely and often with force. Such irritation is usually caused by hidden food allergies and/ or sensitivities. In fact, diarrhea is one of the most common symptoms of food allergy. The colons of some people are so sensitive that they react to some common foods as if they were poisons. The foods implicated vary from person to person, but often include such things as wheat, milk products, oranges and citrus fruit, caffeine (e.g., coffee, tea, colas), and/or the nightshade family (e.g., tomatoes, potatoes, eggplant, peppers, paprika, cayenne, tobacco, chili). Tracking down and eliminating the offending foods usually brings prompt relief. Going part way, however, does not bring full relief. If diarrhea is caused by a hidden food sensitivity, then total relief will not come until every bit of the offending food is eliminated from the diet. A little bit of a poison is still a poison.

Stools which are loose and frothy (as opposed to watery) often indicate some form of intestinal malabsorption. Such stools may contain fats, shreds of mucus and/or bits of recognizable, undigested foods. Whenever absorption is poor, fats tend to pass through the gut, making the stools looser. Mucus is the body's way of protecting delicate tissues from harm. Its presence in the stools indicates that there is irritation and possible damage to either the small or large intestine, or both. Malabsorption is found in such conditions as lactose intolerance, disaccharidase deficiencies, celiac disease, leaky gut syndrome and Crohn's disease.

CONSTIPATION

Constipation results from infrequent or sluggish action of the bowels. Sometimes the stools are dry, hard, compacted and difficult to pass; but often they appear quite normal. Surprisingly, diarrhea can also be a symptom of constipation. Sometimes the stools become so severely compacted that the only waste that can make it through is liquid.

Many people are constipated and don't know it. Try the beet test. Eat some beets and see how long it takes to pass the characteristic deep red stain in the stools. If it is 24 hours or less, then everything is as it should be. If the red color takes longer than one day to pass, then there is some degree of constipation present. If it takes three days or longer, then constipation is a serious threat to health.

During constipation, some of the cellulose in food is broken down by bacterial action into volatile fatty acids. The growth of bacteria increases in the colon and begins to move upward into the small intestine, where food is fermented more and digested less, causing more gas to be produced. Putrefaction in the colon can produce dangerous free-radical generating substances (e.g., apcholic acid, 3-methyl cholanthrene) that have been implicated as causative factors in cancer and arterial disease. Constipated people are also at higher risk for appendicitis, hiatal hernia, diverticulosis, haemorrhoids and varicose veins.

Constipation usually indicates that the body lacks sufficient fiber, water, or both. Drink at least two liters/quarts of purified water daily. Increase dietary fiber by consuming generous amounts of vegetables, 100 percent whole grains, nuts, seeds, and fruits. For good measure, also include regular exercise. Simply walking for 20 minutes each day may be enough to relieve constipation for those with sedentary lifestyles.

Both diarrhea and constipation usually improve by adding more bulk to the stools. A larger, bulkier stool passes through the colon more easily and requires less straining during defecation, thereby reducing the risk of forming diverticula, haemorrhoids and varicose veins. If increasing dietary fiber from food sources is not enough to do the job, then consider taking a natural bulking agent. Finely powdered psyllium (plantago) hulls are most efficient in this respect. One rounded tablespoonful in 10 ounces (300 ml.) of water can make a dramatic difference to normalizing bowel transit time – slowing it down if it is too fast and speeding it up if it is too slow. [Note: *Psyllium is a bulking agent, **not** a laxative. Laxatives work by irritating the colon; psyllium works simply by filling the colon with smooth, gelatinous fiber, as nature intended. Also, psyllium can help to correct diarrhea; no laxative can do that.*]

Both diarrhea and constipation disturb intestinal bacteria, so it is a good idea to help normalize microflora by taking supplementary *Lactobacillus acidophilus.* (Someone who is lactose intolerant needs to take a lactose-free *L. acidophilus*, such as one that is grown on malto-dextrins).

To correct constipation, it is best to start the bowels moving with an herbal laxative before supplementing with psyllium. Then, as movements become more free, reduce the herbal laxative and introduce the psyllium bulking agent on a regular basis. Psyllium is highly absorptive and needs to be taken with lots of water. About three quarts of water daily are required to optimize the effectiveness of psyllium. Omitting the herbal laxative primer and/or having too low a water intake may cause the psyllium to become impacted in the colon, adding to constipation rather than relieving it. It is important to withdraw the herbal laxative when no longer needed. To overuse any laxative (even natural, herbal ones) can create a dependence whereby the bowels become lazy and do not move without it.

Chronic constipation that is not fully relieved by the above may suggest a need for supplementary hydrochloric acid and/or bile, which is a natural laxative. An enzyme supplement containing both of these factors can be most helpful in such cases.

LOW STOMACH ACID

The stomach is a critical link in the chain of digestion. If it functions well, then everything else tends to as well. If it is underactive, then supporting it will benefit the entire digestive tract.

Most children and young adults can usually eat whatever they like, in whatever combination, without experiencing gastric distress. Unfortunately, the older we get, the less hydrochloric acid our stomachs produce. Almost everyone over age 40 can benefit from some kind of digestive support.

Symptoms of low stomach acid include:

- ☐ Excessive gas, belching or burping after meals.
- ☐ Abdominal bloating, distension.
- ☐ Indigestion or sourness two to three hours after eating.
- ☐ Heavy, tired feeling after eating.
- ☐ Burning sensation in the stomach.
- ☐ Full, heavy or lethargic feeling after eating meat.
- ☐ Loss of former taste or craving for meat.
- ☐ Constipation.

Stomach acidity affects every stage of digestion. It activates pepsin, the stomach enzyme that digests proteins. It stimulates the gallbladder to release bile, which emulsifies fats. It triggers the release of the pancreatic enzymes that break down proteins, starches, and fats. Stomach acidity also creates an unfavorable environment for harmful bacteria and parasites.

When the stomach isn't acidic enough (hypochlorhydria), the entire digestive system slows down. Proteins are not broken down into their constituent amino acids. Insufficient bile is released, causing fats to glob together in the gut, attracting minerals to form insoluble soaps. Pancreatic enzymes are not released in sufficient quantity to break the food mass into small enough particles to pass through the intestinal wall, thus hindering absorption. Intestinal immunity suffers because the population of beneficial flora becomes displaced by putrefactive by-products of incomplete digestion. Colon function and elimination stagnate. Toxins are released in the gut, some of which may be absorbed into the bloodstream.

Some people have learned to avoid the foods that are difficult for them to digest, but such an approach may deprive them of much needed protein and other factors. A far better way is to support the digestive weaknesses.

Sometimes the simple practise of separating proteins and sugars is enough to restore complete digestion. Where this guideline is consistently applied without full results, then further help is needed. Some people find varying degrees of relief from taking a very dilute drink of apple cider vinegar before a meal or by consuming acidic foods with the meal (e.g., sauerkraut, pickles, vinaigrette dressings). For most, however, such aids are but a small step in the right direction.

DIGESTIVE SUPPORT

The best way to improve digestion is to support all of the interdependent links in the digestive chain. The following is a sample of a digestive enzyme formula that does just that. The amounts given are for a single tablet. One may take one or more tablets with each meal that is difficult to digest: **betaine hydrochloride** (88 mg.), **pepsin** 1:3,000 (110 mg.), **pancreatin** 8X (28 mg.), **bile** (88 mg.), **bromelain** (44 mg.), **papain** 12M (122 mg.), **peppermint** (66 mg.).

Taking the above digestive aid immediately after each meal is the preferred way. Doing so encourages the body do what it can on its own, then follows up with support for what it cannot do. Taking the enzymes before the meal may encourage dependence on them; the body may get lazy and stop producing what it does not have to.

In the above formula, betaine hydrochloride provides the hydrochloric acid needed to activate pepsin and to sterilize the stomach from bacteria and parasites. Pepsin is the stomach's proteolytic enzyme. Pancreatin provides protease, amylase and lipase enzymes. Bile emulsifies fats, sterilizes the intestines from putrefaction and parasites, and acts as a laxative. Papain is a proteolytic enzyme found in raw papaya. Its inclusion in this supplement can enhance the action of pepsin and the pancreatic protease. Peppermint is an herbal carminative. It soothes the intestinal tract and helps to remove gas.

There is an art to knowing how many digestive enzyme tablets to take. Requirements differ from person to person. Also, the same person's needs can change from day to day, depending on the type, quantity and combinations of foods eaten and one's stress level at the time of eating. Some people start with one tablet per meal to see how much improvement there is, then continue adding more tablets at future meals (of similar composition) until there is no more gas or discomfort. With a little experimentation one may find, for example, that a meal containing only fruit, a salad or a light soup would not require any digestive enzyme tablets. A typical breakfast might require one tablet, lunch two, dinner three.

Another way to find an optimal daily level is to take one enzyme complex tablet on an empty stomach, first thing in the morning after rising.

The second morning take two tablets on an empty stomach. The third morning take three, and so on. Continue adding one tablet per morning until a burning sensation is felt in the stomach. If that occurs at say, seven tablets, then reduce that number by one (i.e., to six) and that will be the number of tablets to take on a *daily* basis, in divided amounts with meals (e.g., two per meal).

A word of caution: Enzyme formulas containing hydrochloric acid (e.g., betaine hydrochloride. glutamic acid hydrochloride) should not be taken if there is an ulcer present.

Without adequate supplies of hydrochloric acid, pepsin and pancreatic enzymes, the body cannot adequately break down protein into its constituent amino acids. These amino acids, in turn, are the building blocks of every cell in our bodies. They are also needed to build antibodies, hormones and enzymes. Here we have a "catch-22" situation: if our bodies do not produce enough digestive enzymes, they cannot break down protein sufficiently to produce more of those same enzymes. Taking supplementary enzymes can help to break this cycle.

METABOLIC LIMITATIONS

Some people's bodies do not produce all of the enzymes necessary to digest all of the food factors that are provided by a typical healthy diet. Some may be born without certain enzymes; others may lose them as they get older. Biochemically, each of us is unique. The following are examples of digestive and health problems created by missing links in the chain of digestive enzymes.

LACTOSE INTOLERANCE

It is nature's plan that young mammals consume mother's milk until they are able to feed themselves. Once they have been weaned to solid food, however, they never drink milk again. The enzyme, lactase, that their intestines needed to break down lactose (milk sugar) is no longer required; and so their bodies stop producing it.

Humans are included in this mammalian plan. Once our digestive systems have fully matured, there is no biological necessity for us to continue to drink milk. With some cultural exceptions, humans also lose the ability to produce lactase.

Humans differ from other mammals in that (1) we consume milk beyond the weaning period, and (2) we drink the milk of other species. Some humans are better able than others to adapt to the extended consumption of milk. If we drink it into our adult life, we may or may not be able to continue to produce lactase. It depends on both our inherited tendencies and how frequently we ingest milk products. Some genetically weak infants are born without the ability to produce lactase at all. Those who can produce it often lose the ability in later childhood or early adulthood. Some individuals retain the ability to produce lactase their entire lives. It is a matter of biochemical individuality.

Lactose intolerance can be primary if it happens spontaneously – or secondary, if caused by deterioration of the microvilli in the small intestine caused by celiac sprue or Crohn's disease. Many people who are lactose intolerant are totally so; their bodies do not produce any lactase at all. Although they may not have any overt symptoms until they reach a certain level of milk intake daily, even tiny amounts of lactose can impair their digestive ability. For that reason, total abstinence from milk products is highly recommended. It makes no difference if the milk product is from a cow or a goat; the milk of all species contains lactose.

Most of the world's adult population have lost the ability to produce lactase in their intestines. Lactase deficiency (or lactose intolerance) may affect from 70 to 95 percent of those of Asian, African, Native American and Mediterranean descent – and from 15 to 25 percent of those of Scandinavian and Anglo-Saxon descent.

In those descended from Northern European stock where dairying has been practised for centuries, only about 20 percent appear to be lactose intolerant. In the African-American population, lactase deficiency is estimated to be about 80 percent in adults and 35 percent in children under age 11. The prevalence of lactase deficiency may be 100 percent in Asian adults living in the U.S., and over 50 percent in Mexican Americans. Native Americans and Alaskan Inuit have been found to be about 95 percent lactose intolerant.

In some parts of India and Africa where dairying and milk consumption have continued for thousands of years, about 20 percent or less of the adults have difficulty digesting lactose. In pastoral tribes in these same countries, however, where milk is not used after infancy, lactose intolerance is seen in about 80 percent of adults. In most ethnic groups where milk drinking is not traditional, the lactase enzyme disappears at about the time of weaning. On a worldwide basis, this is the norm. In America, white children are expected to have normal lactase activity until at least five years of age and black children until only three years of age.

Lactose intolerance results from the absence of lactase in the microvilli of the small intestine. Consequently, lactose (a disaccharide) cannot be broken down into its monosaccharide components, glucose and galactose. Lactose then stays in the intestinal tract, fermenting and feeding certain bacteria that produce large amounts of methane, carbon dioxide and hydrogen gases, causing flatulence and abdominal discomfort. The lactose and its bacterially formed metabolites retain water in the gut, which can result in cramps and diarrhea. Symptoms may range from mild abdominal discomfort and bloating to severe diarrhea from consuming even very small amounts of lactose.

Continued consumption of milk products by those with lactose intolerance tends to produce fatigue and a predisposition to catch colds, bronchitis and ear infections. How many symptoms and to what degree a person has them is very much an individual matter. Sometimes in those who have otherwise strong constitutions, the only noticeable symptom of lactose intolerance is chronic fatigue.

One way to find out if you have a lactase deficiency is to take a lactose tolerance test. This laboratory procedure involves measuring the amount of galactose in the blood after drinking a solution containing lactose. A simpler method is to stop consuming all milk products for at least two weeks to see if symptoms diminish or disappear.

Anyone who has a lactose intolerance is well advised to avoid all dairy products (e.g., milk, buttermilk, cheese, cottage cheese, ice cream, yogurt) and all foods with lactose, whey, or milk solids as a hidden ingredient. Yogurt that is homemade or cultured after it was pasteurized may have about 70 percent less lactose than that found in the equivalent amount of milk. This is because the lactic bacteria in yogurt break down some of its lactose content. Some people are able to tolerate the small amount of lactose in yogurt; many cannot. Similarly, some cheeses contain less lactose than others.

The one dairy product that most lactose intolerant people can safely consume is butter, which may contain only minute traces of lactose. Even this tiny bit of lactose can be completely removed by clarifying the butter to make ghee.

Lactose free cheeses are a safe bet. During the cheese making process, most of the lactose is drained off with the whey. The small amount that remains is changed to lactic acid during the ripening (aging) process. The longer the cheese is aged, the less lactose remains. The following cheeses characteristically have from a zero to two percent lactose content: muenster, edam, camembert, brie, provolone, cheddar (sharp), and gouda. By monitoring lactose content, manufacturers can produce various forms of these and other cheeses that are totally lactose free.

Milk promoted as being lactose free is a different story. This is because the lactase enzymes added to the milk are harvested from bacteria and fungi, which produce their lactase to be efficient under conditions of temperature and acidity that may differ from those found in commercially produced milk. The trace amounts of lactose remaining in so-called lactose free milk can be problematic to those who are highly sensitive to it.

There are also a number of lactase enzyme supplements available – tablets or capsules that one takes when consuming dairy products. These have the same limitation as above, namely that the lactase they provide is harvested from bacteria and fungi, rather than from mammals. Experiment to see how well these products may work for you.

The dairy industry and dieticians would have us believe that we cannot get enough calcium without consuming dairy products. Not so. The cows that provide calcium-rich milk don't drink milk themselves. They have incredibly strong bones and enough calcium left over to put into their milk supply. Cows get all of the calcium they need from the grasses and grains that they eat. The same is true of adult mammals of all species. Osteoporosis and osteomalacia are unknown among all animals consuming the food that is natural to them. Calcium is widely dispersed in nature. Most of us can get all we need from a varied diet that includes generous amounts of such foods as soybeans/tofu, sardines, salmon, peanuts, walnuts, sunflower seeds, dried beans, green vegetables, almonds and beef liver. Like our paleolithic ancestors, food foragers in primitive cultures consume over 2,000 mg. of calcium daily without ingesting a single lick or smell of any milk product.

Sometimes the diet may not provide enough calcium for a particular person's needs. In such cases, the lactose intolerant person would be far better to take a calcium supplement than to consume a substance that her body does not need and cannot handle. For the fortunate minority who can tolerate lactose, milk products can be quite nourishing. The majority of adults, however, can become ill by consuming them.

DISACCHARIDASE DEFICIENCIES

The healthy intestinal wall produces disaccharidase enzymes that break down lactose, sucrose, maltose, and isomaltose into simple sugars (monosaccharides). Lactose and sucrose exist as sugars in various foods. Maltose and isomaltose are intermediate sugars that result from the breakdown of starches by amylase enzymes.

Damage to the mucosal cells of the small intestine can impair its ability to produce disaccharidases. Such damage may be caused by acute illnesses (e.g., bacterial infections, diarrhea), by gluten enteropathy (celiac disease), by chronic food allergies, or by overuse of some prescription drugs.

Without adequate disaccharidases, undigested carbohydrates remain in the intestinal tract, fermenting and producing excess gas. Unabsorbed carbohydrates also provide excellent food for undesirable bacteria. They encourage microbes from the colon to take up residence and multiply in the small intestine, where they do not belong. This kind of bacterial growth in the small intestine may damage its microvilli and further suppress the production of disaccharidases. In order to protect its delicate lining from such damage, the small intestine secretes extra amounts of mucus, which has the effect of reducing absorption even further.

Any substance that irritates the small intestine – including allergens and bacteria – cause its delicate lining to lay down mucus that is much thicker than normal. This excessive mucus restricts food particles from reaching the enzymes in the microvilli. Thus, a person may be producing adequate amounts of disaccharidases but still not be able to digest disaccharides because of the mucus barrier.

Carbohydrate not absorbed by the body but metabolized by bacteria gives off hydrogen. Therefore, disaccharidase deficiencies (including lactose intolerance) can be diagnosed by measurement of hydrogen gas in exhaled breath. (This test is only reliable for finding disaccharidase deficiencies if done more than 48 hours after eating beans, the digestion of which also releases hydrogen.)

Disaccharidase deficiencies are usually self-correcting, once the small intestine has healed and intestinal flora have returned to normal. A major exception to the above is lactase, whose absence is permanent in large numbers of people for genetic reasons. (In some cases, however, a lactase deficiency may be only temporarily induced by infection or by some other food sensitivity.) Another exception is hereditary sucrase deficiency, which has been found in about 10 percent of Greenland Inuit and is estimated to affect about two percent of North Americans.

Intestinal tissue is self-regenerative. In time, it will heal itself – if and only if there is total abstinence from all of the foods and other substances that irritate it. In the case of disaccharidase deficiencies, it is necessary to eliminate (1) all dairy products (e.g., milk, cheese, cottage cheese, yogurt, ice cream), (2) all grains (e.g., wheat, rye, oats, barley, corn, rice, buckwheat, millet, triticale, bulgur, spelt, kamut, quinoa, amaranth, couscous), (3) all starchy vegetables and legumes (e.g., potatoes, yams, sweet potatoes, parsnips, beets, carrots, pumpkin, squash, turnips, dried beans, soybeans, chickpeas, lentils, peas, carob,), and (4) all sources of sucrose (table sugar, molasses, maple sugar, corn syrup).

Strict adherence to this low-disaccharide diet means preparing every meal from fresh or frozen foods. Processed and canned foods are notorious for including hidden flours, starches and sugars. Acceptable foods include meat, poultry, fish, eggs, nuts, and low-starch vegetables (e.g., asparagus, broccoli, Brussels sprouts, cabbage, cauliflower, celery, cucumbers, eggplant, garlic, kale, lettuce, mushrooms, onions, parsley, spinach, string beans, tomatoes, watercress). Fruits, fruit juices (preferably dilute), and honey (used sparingly) are also acceptable, since the sugars they provide are primarily monosaccharides (fructose and glucose) that are absorbed directly through the intestinal wall.

Total abstinence from everything that is irritating the lining of the small intestine enables that tissue to repair itself. Disaccharide deficiencies are often secondary to something else. If they are caused entirely by acute inflammation, then following the low disaccharide diet may enable the small intestine to repair itself within two weeks or so of eliminating the causative bacteria or virus. If the primary cause is chronic or multifactorial (e.g., from candidiasis, hidden food allergies, drug reactions), then full recovery of disaccharidase production may take up to three months or so on the low-disaccharide diet, depending on how diligent one has been in tracking down and eliminating the primary cause(s). If it takes longer than this for complete recovery, then there are two possibilities: Either (1) not all of the primary causative factors have been eliminated, or (2) one has not been vigilant enough in following the diet. Including even small amounts of yogurt, low-lactose cheeses, and starchy vegetables can significantly reduce the effectiveness of the low-disaccharide diet. A little bit of a poison is still a poison, so to speak.

Some people are tempted to cut corners by taking supplementary enzyme complexes that contain disaccharidases (i.e., sucrase or invertase, maltase, isomaltase, lactase). Doing so enables the body to break down some of the disaccharides ingested. Such supplements are a good emergency aid to have when one must eat something and there are no disaccharide-free foods available. To try to rely on them on a regular basis, however, could be unreliable. To match the exact quantities of these enzymes required to varying quantities and kinds of sugars consumed is very difficult, on a meal by meal basis. Some disaccharides are bound to slip through.

The low-disaccharide diet is a demanding one to follow. Fortunately, the necessity to do so is usually only temporary. The more strictly one adheres to it, the faster recovery will be. Total results require a total commitment.

Some people feel so good on the low-saccharide diet that they choose to follow it for life. This is a very healthy way to eat. Ninety-five percent of all human beings who have ever lived were (or still are) food foragers. They live(d) free of most degenerative diseases by consuming only wild game, fish, bird's eggs, green leafy plants, nuts, seeds, berries and fruits – *no* milk products, *no* grains, *no* table sugar, and *no* processed foods of any kind.

When to end the low-disaccharide diet is a judgment call. If the original problem was chronic, it is not good to come off the diet until one has been symptom-free for at least one month. At that time one can experiment by adding a small amount of a grain or other starch at one meal on a particular day. Wait for four more days, then have another starchy food. Wait for three days, then try again, and again after two more days. For the next two weeks, alternate by having one grain or starch at only one meal on every second day. If any gastrointestinal symptoms recur at any time during this re-introduction program, it means that healing is not complete and the low-saccharide diet needs to be resumed. If no symptoms are produced, then it is probably safe to resume consuming moderate amounts of grains/ starches on a daily basis.

FAVISM

Favism is a rare hereditary condition, common in Sicily and Sardinia, that causes a sensitivity to a species of bean, *Vicia faba*. It is characterized by fever, acute haemolytic anemia, vomiting, diarrhea, and may lead to prostration and coma. It is caused by an inherited deficiency of the enzyme, glucose-6-phosphate dehydrogenase. Although this a rare form of food intolerance, it is included here as an example to show that just about any enzyme deficiency may be possible.

GLUTEN INTOLERANCE

Gluten is vegetable albumin, the main protein found in wheat, rye, oats, barley, and related grains. It is composed of glutenin and gliadin, the factor responsible for the sticky mass that results when wheat flour and water are mixed. In some individuals, however, the intestinal mucosa lacks the ability to digest gliadin, allowing it to damage the lining. This is a gluten-induced form of enteropathy that is usually referred to as celiac sprue. It is a deterioration of the intestinal tract characterized by malabsorption, weight loss, abdominal distension, bloating, and steatorrhea (increased secretion of fat from the sebaceous glands of the skin).

Some babies are born with a genetic weakness that makes them totally gluten intolerant. These celiac infants experience malnutrition, weight loss, muscle wasting, abdominal distension, irritability, loss of muscle tone, and retarded motor development. Older celiac children tend to develop behavioral problems, anemia, rickets, and multiple vitamin and mineral deficiencies.

Much of the time, gluten sensitivity seems to be acquired rather than inherited. It usually appears during the first three years. Introducing cow's milk and cereals into the infant's diet too early may be causative factors. Breastfed babies have a lower risk of developing celiac disease. Sometimes, however, the problem does not appear until a person is in her twenties.

In full blown celiac disease, the stools tend to be bulky, soft, pale, frothy, foul-smelling, greasy and frequent. Undigested gliadin actually destroys the villi and microvilli in the small intestine, significantly reducing its absorptive surface and creating chronic intestinal malabsorption. Incomplete protein metabolites are absorbed into the bloodstream where they may affect the immune system and alter brain chemistry. Behavioral abnormalities, mental confusion, poor memory and schizophrenia are more common among celiacs than among the general population.

Clinical diagnosis of a celiac condition is based on the intestinal damage it causes. A biopsy of the jejunum is taken. If the microvilli are missing or flattened, then the person has celiac disease. It the microvilli are healthy, then s/he does not. (A much less invasive way to diagnose the condition is simply to eliminate gluten from the diet entirely for at least two weeks. If symptoms disappear, then gluten intolerance is their most likely cause.)

Gliadin that has been pre-digested does not activate celiac disease in susceptible people. Therefore, the most likely explanation for a gluten sensitivity is that the individual lacks the enzyme necessary to break down gliadin into simpler peptides. Humans in general have been consuming cultivated grains for about 10,000 years or so, and in some cultures for only about 3,000 years. (For well over 50,000 years they ate only meat, fish, vegetables, fruits, nuts and seeds.) Thus, genetically speaking, humans have had a relatively short time to adapt to this new source of food. Some individuals still are not able to produce the enzyme necessary to handle it.

The celiac individual needs to eliminate from the diet all grains that contain gluten – including wheat, kamut, rye, triticale, spelt, barley and oats (unless these grains are 100 per sprouted, which process breaks down the gliadin.) One needs to be vigilant about wheat flour, a hidden ingredient in many processed foods. Abstinence from these foods must be total. It is another case of a little bit of a poison is still a poison. Acceptable grain substitutes that do not contain gluten include rice, corn (maize), millet, amaranth, quinoa and buckwheat. The damage caused by gliadin also impairs the intestine's ability to produce lactase. Therefore, most celiacs are also lactose intolerant and need to eliminate all milk products as well. Total abstinence from both gluten and lactose may reduce celiac symptoms significantly within five days to two weeks. If it does not, then other disaccharidase deficiencies may be involved and the person may also have to follow the low-disaccharide diet described previously. Total remission of symptoms may take several months, depending on individual response.

Avoidance is not cure, however. Dietary relapses bring a recurrence of symptoms. That is because the inability to digest gluten is a genetic weakness that cannot be revived by dietary, nutritional or medical means. In true celiac disease, following the gluten-free diet is a lifelong necessity.

(If the celiac condition has also induced disaccharidase deficiencies, however, then these may recover as the small intestine heals itself.)

Because of intestinal malabsorption, every celiac will have also multiple nutrient deficiencies. Thus, it is most beneficial to take a high-potency, broad-spectrum vitamin-mineral supplement. Doing so will both speed the recovery process and help to correct both marginal and long standing deficiencies.

CROHN'S DISEASE

Crohn's disease (regional ileitis, regional enteritis) involves chronic non-specific inflammation of the lowest part of the small intestine. Symptoms may come and go and include diarrhea, abdominal pain, anemia, weight loss, fistula formation, and eventual intestinal blockage. Stools are soft and gray or brown in color, with abnormal fecal particles.

Crohn's disease is a reaction to hidden food allergies. The most likely culprits are gluten (wheat, rye, oats, barley, triticale) and milk products (lactose). There may also be sensitivities to soy, egg, nuts, and/or the nightshades (tomatoes, potatoes, peppers, paprika, eggplant, cayenne, chili).

Complete recovery from Crohn's disease is possible if and only if all of the offending foods are totally eliminated. A little bit of a poison is still a poison, so to speak. Eating even tiny amounts of the offenders will cause a return of the disease. Recovery from Crohn's is also facilitated by a high fiber, low sugar diet – but the fiber must be from non-glutinous sources (e.g., vegetables, brown rice, buckwheat, amaranth).

Because of inefficient absorption, those with Crohn's disease tend to be deficient in the fat-soluble vitamins (A, D, E), the B-complex vitamins (especially B-12 & folic acid), calcium, magnesium, iron, selenium, and zinc.

WHEAT SENSITIVITY

Many who can digest gluten have a low tolerance to wheat itself. It is not the gluten in the wheat that is the problem but some other factor(s).

Wheat is the agricultural crop that has been most affected by humans' desire to change nature. It has been hybridized and genetically engineered to alter its chromosomes. Wheat crops are also heavily laden with agricultural chemicals, the full effects of which on human health are unknown. The attempt to develop a commercially successful staple have, unfortunately, rendered it indigestible by large numbers of people.

Gluten tolerant people who have difficulty digesting wheat can usually handle kamut and spelt, two ancient wheat-like grains overlooked by food tinkering scientists. Even those who are tolerant of wheat would be do well to limit their consumption of it to the equivalent of two slices of bread daily. Organic whole grain wheat is far preferable to any of its commercial counterparts.

GUIDELINES FOR HEALTHY DIGESTION

Following is a summary of guidelines that help to create optimal conditions for digestion. They allow one's natural processes of digestion, absorption, elimination and intestinal immunity to work as efficiently as possible.

TIMING

- Eat only when genuinely hungry.
- Have the largest meal in the middle of the day.
- Rest briefly before and after each meal.
- Spend at least 30 minutes eating each meal.
- Allow 3 hours between meals.
- Consume nothing after 9 PM.

SETTING THE MOOD

- Do not eat when angry, anxious, upset or overtired.
- Begin each meal quietly, with a silent pause.
- Eat with congenial company in pleasant conversation, or
- Eat alone in contemplative silence or with pleasant music.
- Avoid reading, watching TV or arguing while eating.

AWARENESS

- Eat slowly, chewing food thoroughly.
- Take time to enjoy tastes, textures and aromas.

- Imagine food being transformed into your bodily cells.
- Swallow only when each mouthful has turned to paste.
- Eat only enough to feel good. Never stuff yourself.

INFANTS

- Nurse infants for as long as possible (up to 24 months).
- First solid foods: pureed meats, green vegetables, fruits.
- No cereals or starchy foods until infant has molars.

FOOD SELECTION

- Drink two plus litres of purified water daily.
- Large amounts of dietary fiber (unrefined plant foods).
- Avoid processed foods, refined sugars and flours.
- Consume alcohol and caffeine sparingly, if at all.
- Suspect allergy/intolerance to any food that one craves.
- Observe body's reactions to lactose, gluten and wheat.

FOOD COMBINING

- No sugars with proteins or fats at the same meal.
- Fruits/juices 30 minutes before or 3 hours after meals.
- Sip water when mouth is empty or at the end of a meal.

SUPPLEMENTS

- Take vitamin-mineral supplements with meals.
- Support digestion with supplementary enzymes.

GALLBLADDER PROBLEMS

There are two kinds of gallbladder problems. One is inflammation of the gallbladder (cholecystitis), often caused by hidden food allergies that cause the cystic duct to go into spasm. The other and more usual is cholelithiasis (gallstones). whereby bilestones or calculi form in the gallbladder or common duct.

Bile is the digestive agent that controls gas resulting from the fermentation of carbohydrates, and from the putrefaction of proteins and the bacteria that feed on them. Bile does nothing to digest either carbohydrates or proteins, but it does have a sterilizing effect on fermentation and putrefactive bacteria. Insufficient bile causes gas to accumulate in both upper and lower intestines.

The following are symptoms of gallbladder problems:

☐ consistent gas and bloating from most foods
☐ fats/greasy foods cause nausea or headaches
☐ onions, cabbage, radishes, cucumbers cause bloating
☐ skin oily on nose and forehead
☐ constipation
☐ bad breath or bad taste in mouth
☐ excess body odor
☐ stools yellow or clay colored

Medical symptoms of gallbladder restriction include pain in the upper abdomen, pain referred to the back or right shoulder, and sometimes mild jaundice. The nutritional tipoff before it gets this far is to notice if almost every food or meal causes bloating.

Consistent bloating indicates that insufficient bile is being excreted into the duodenum. Some or all of the following foods may cause digestive difficulty: Brussels sprouts, cabbage, cucumbers, curry, garlic, onions, radishes, sauerkraut, turnips. Most fatty foods will be difficult to digest and may cause considerable discomfort, with the possible exception of butter. (The fat in butter is pre-emulsified and so does not require bile. It is largely broken down by gastric lipase before it reaches the duodenum.)

Sometimes food allergies or may cause gallbladder attacks in sensitive people. Ingesting allergy-causing substances may cause swelling of the bile duct, resulting in restricted bile flow from the gallbladder. One study found that 100 percent of a group of patients were free from gallbladder attacks while they were on a hypoallergenic diet (consisting of beef, rye, soybeans, rice, cherry, peach, apricot, beet and spinach). Foods most likely to induce gallbladder pain in sensitive people, according to this study, were egg, pork, onion, poultry, milk, coffee, citrus fruit, corn, beans and nuts.

These four steps help the liver and gallbladder to supply bile in sufficient quantity and with the proper flow characteristics: (1) drink at least two litres of water daily, (2) increase dietary fiber (vegetables, whole grains, fruits), (3) avoid all sugars and fried foods, (4) increase consumption of olive oil, and (5) take the following supplements daily: **vitamin C** (2,000 mg.), **vitamin E** (400 I.U.), **lecithin** (1,200 mg.), and at least 5 grams of finely powdered **psyllium** hulls in a large glass of water.

CHOLECYSTECTOMY

Cholecystectomy is surgical removal of the gallbladder. The gallbladder stores bile produced by the liver and concentrates it up to four times its original strength, keeping it in a sac ready to be squirted into the duodenum as needed to emulsify fats. Without a gallbladder, a weaker form of bile trickles into the duodenum – and there is none on reserve to match the timing of most dietary fats. The result is that fats enter the small intestine in globules too large to be broken down by lipase enzymes. These undigested fats attract minerals (by opposing electromagnetic charges) to form insoluble soaps, which are constipating. Neither the fats nor the minerals are absorbed. During constipation, free radicals are produced. Anyone without a gallbladder is thus at increased risk for colon cancer and degenerative conditions related to mineral deficiencies (e.g., osteoporosis).

Anyone without a gallbladder needs continuing digestive support. Without this important organ, there is no way that bile released into the duodenum will be enough (either in strength or quantity) to do the job required. Constipation, poor mineral absorption and a greater risk for colon cancer may be the result. The solution is simple, however: take a digestive aid containing bile salts with each meal that contains fats or would otherwise cause discomfort.

GALLSTONES

When the flow of bile is too slow and too much concentrating takes place in the gallbladder, stones are often formed. Some of these stones can become stuck in the bile duct and cause a back pressure known as gallbladder colic.

Most gallstones consist of crystals of cholesterol, bile acids, bile pigments, and sometimes calcium and other substances. Diets high in sugars and refined flour tend to produce bile that is more supersaturated with cholesterol (and thus more likely to form stones) than diets high in fiber. The incidence of gallstones is also higher when polyunsaturated oils are the predominant source of dietary fats, and lower when monounsaturates (e.g., olive oil) are consumed liberally. Low stomach acid may also contribute to gallbladder involvement, because if hydrochloric acid levels are low, the gall bladder does not receive the proper pH signals to trigger a sufficient release of bile when required, thus allowing bile to accumulate and stagnate.

Once stones have formed, therapeutic measures may be required to remove them. The medical approach is to remove the entire gallbladder, an extremely important part of one's digestive anatomy and physiology. There is, however, a far less drastic method that does not require sacrificing this vital organ.

GALLBLADDER FLUSH

The following is a safe, simple and time-tested method of passing gallstones that has been used by many thousands of people for decades. (1) For three days consume three to four litres per day of apple juice or cider, and no other food or liquid (except water, if desired). (2) Mix two tablespoons of finely powdered psyllium hulls into 10 ounces of the allotted apple juice (or water) and drink this down – once on the first day, twice on the second day, three times on the third day. (3) On the evening of the first and second days, mix two ounces (60 mL) of pure, extra virgin olive oil and two ounces (60 mL) of freshly squeezed lemon juice thoroughly and drink this mixture down. (4) On the evening of the third day, repeat step #3, but this time double the quantities of olive oil and lemon juice to 4 ounces (120 mL) each.

The stones soften and begin to pass after the third day, and sometimes sooner. Stones up to 0.75 inch (2 cm.) in diameter have been observed to pass in the stools in this manner; however, it is more usual to get a shower of 100 or more tiny ones at a time. In some cases, the stones may dissolve before reaching the stools and are not observable.

There is a theoretical risk to the above procedure, although it has never been reported. If a stone were to become wedged in the bile duct during the flushing, it would have to be removed surgically – from the duct, not the gallbladder. To my knowledge, surgical intervention has never been required as a result of this gallbladder flush; however, it is a consideration to keep in mind. If it were to happen, one could come through the experience with one's gallbladder still intact (to the extent that you are able to convince the surgeon not to remove a healthy gallbladder.)

ONE'S FOOD IS ANOTHER'S POISON

The title of this chapter is paraphrased from Hippocrates (460-361 BC): *"What is meat [i.e., food] to one person can be fierce poison to another."* Hippocrates is also reputed to have said, *"To many this has been the commencement of a serious disease when they have merely taken twice in a day the same food that they have been in the custom of taking once."* One of his earliest dietary observations was that milk could cause gastric upset and hives in sensitive people. Today's physicians would do well to note that hidden food sensitivities could be the leading cause of most undiagnosed symptoms.

There is no food that is ideal for everyone. There is no diet that brings health to all. What are the best foods for a particular individual depend on that person's unique biochemistry.

Foods considered healthy for the general population can behave like slow poisons in those who have sensitivities to them. Tofu, yogurt, granola, wheat germ, whole grain breads – oatmeal, milk, eggs, orange juice, broccoli – all of these fine foods actually make some people sick. It is hard to believe that a simple matter of food choice can have devastating consequences. Health advocates are sometimes the hardest to convince, especially those who fervently believe in a "one diet fits all" approach.

Undiagnosed food sensitivities affect more than half of the population. Almost everyone has at least one sensitivity. Many are not aware, however, that their symptoms are caused by inappropriate food choices. They continue to eat the same foods, day after day, never getting complete relief from supplements or lifestyle changes. Unaware that their favorite foods are undermining their health, some bounce from practitioner to practitioner, only to be labelled hypochondriac.

Unless you are specifically looking for food sensitivities, you are unlikely to find them. Sometimes their symptoms are not directly observable. They may not be the kind of symptoms that show up on allergy testing or they may be in parts of the body not exposed to view, such as the early tissue changes that lead to arthritis, Crohn's disease or schizophrenia. Sensitivity reactions are also not often recognized for what they are. That is because they are such great masqueraders. They can mimic almost any ailment and affect almost any organ or tissue in the body.

Food sensitivities are of two basic kinds: allergies and intolerances. An allergy is an unnatural immune reaction to a specific protein in a food that is otherwise harmless to most people. The body builds antibodies to these foreign proteins, and the skirmish between antibody and invader produces side effects wherein nearby tissues become damaged. An intolerance, on the other hand, is an inability of the body to digest or metabolize a particular food constituent, due to overloading it with more than it can handle. Intolerances thus have to do with metabolism rather than immunity. They are usually the consequence of the body's inability to produce a particular digestive enzyme.

If you are allergic to a particular food you will have a zero tolerance for it. You will not be able to consume any amount of it without triggering an unnatural response in your body. You can also have a zero tolerance to a substance for reasons other than allergy. Reactions due entirely to intolerance do not involve immune responses, however; no antibodies are produced to the offending food factors.

Allergies are absolute. You are either allergic to a substance or you are not. Tolerance can be a question of degree, however. If your body produces a little bit of lactase, for example, you may be able to consume small amounts of milk or cheese occasionally with no ill effects. If your body does not produce any lactase at all, you will have a zero tolerance to lactose (milk sugar) in any form. (Judging the degree of intolerance by symptoms alone is a tricky business. Someone with a total lactose intolerance may not have any obvious symptoms until a certain threshold of intake has been reached only because a thicker layer of mucus protecting the intestines tends to dull milder adverse reactions.)

Sometimes it is important to distinguish between allergy and intolerance. In many cases, however, the bottom line is the same regardless of which classification we use. If your body's functioning is in any way impaired by an offending food, then you need to stop eating it.

ALMOST ANY SYMPTOM

The most tell-tale sign of food sensitivity is chronic fatigue – not the usual sort, but an almost painful tiredness that is not helped by bed rest. No matter how much sleep one has, one never feels rested.

In addition to chronic fatigue, just about any other symptom can be also caused by food sensitivities. There are, however, some common threads. These include fluid leakage, muscle spasms, excess mucus, low resistance to infection, poor absorption of nutrients, generalized toxicity, and problems in "target" organs. These are organs in the body uniquely susceptible to attack because of a person's genetic weaknesses or biochemical individuality. These vulnerable organs are the most likely to store toxins and least likely to receive all of the nutrients they need. A sensitivity to a particular food might result, for example, in bladder spasms, a spastic colon, spasm in the throat, or spasms in the neck or back. Sometimes the brain is a target organ, resulting in psychological and behavioral symptoms.

The common cold affects allergy-prone people more than the general population. Some people rarely get colds – the ones who are blessed with strong immune systems unaffected by the foods they eat. Those who succumb to every cold and flu bug going around, however, are usually struggling with undetected food sensitivities. Chronic food reactions weaken their immune systems, lowering their resistance to upper respiratory infections. In a sense, we don't catch colds, we "eat" them. Eliminating the troublesome foods makes colds a thing of the past.

The following is a list of symptoms that can be caused by food allergies and intolerances. This list is incredibly diverse because people are so different biochemically. Some of these symptoms are generalized ones caused by an overworked immune system. Others are specific and relate to which organs or bodily systems are under attack, depending on one's unique vulnerabilities. Almost all of these symptoms can have other possible causes as well. Those followed by an asterisk, however, are ones that are most commonly related to food sensitivities. Also, the more symptoms one has on the entire list, the more likely it is that hidden food reactions are at work.

GENERAL

- Chronic "painful" fatigue*
- Awaken not feeling rested*
- Fatigue not helped by rest*
- Food addictions/cravings*
- Swollen lymph glands*
- Chronic infections*
- Chronic, minor complaints

APPEARANCE

- Dark circles under the eyes*
- Puffiness under the eyes*
- Horizontal creases in lower eyelids*
- Swollen face
- Pale, sallow appearance
- Fluid retention (edema)

GASTROINTESTINAL

- Chronic diarrhea*
- Intestinal malabsorption*
- Spastic colon*
- Irritable bowel*
- Colitis, ulcerative colitis*
- Itchy anus (anal pruritus)
- Loose, frothy stools
- Mucus in stools
- Abdominal bloating/pain
- Heartburn
- Indigestion
- Nervous stomach
- Belching
- Flatulence
- Nausea
- Vomiting

- Constipation
- Gallbladder problems
- Repeating a taste
- Ulcers (gastric or duodenal)
- Gastritis

RESPIRATORY

- Catch colds easily*
- Anaphylactic shock*
- Coughing up phlegm
- Night coughs
- Asthma
- Bronchitis
- Hay fever
- Mucus in bronchial tubes
- Pneumonia
- Wheezing
- Difficulty breathing
- Shortness of breath
- Emphysema

CARDIOVASCULAR

- High blood pressure (hypertension)
- Increased pulse rate
- Heart palpitations
- Rapid heartbeat (tachycardia)
- Irregular heartbeat (arrhythymia)
- Inflammation of veins (phlebitis)
- Inflammation of blood/lymph vessels (vasculitis)
- Blueish or reddish hands
- Hot flashes
- Flushing
- Faintness
- Night sweats
- Swelling of ankles or calves

GENITOURINARY

- Bed-wetting, uncontrolled urination (enuresis)*
- Frequent urination
- Painful urination
- Burning on urination
- Chronic bladder infections
- Vaginal discharge
- Genital itching or pain

MUSCULO-SKELETAL

- Chiropractic adjustments do not last*
- Stiff neck
- Backache
- Muscle spasms
- Muscle cramps
- Muscle pain
- Muscle stiffness or soreness
- Muscle weakness
- Painful, stiff or swollen joints (arthritis)

SKIN

- Hives or welts (urticaria)*
- Eczema*
- Psoriasis*
- Adult acne
- Inflamed, itchy (dermatitis)
- Burning
- Flushing
- Tingling
- Excessive sweating

EYES

- Itching
- Burning
- Red, bloodshot
- Sensitivity to bright lights
- Sandy or gritty feeling
- Excessive watering
- Spots, floaters
- Blurring of vision
- Inflamed iris (iritis)
- Eyelids twitching, itching, or drooping
- Puffy eyelids

NOSE

- Dripping, runny
- Nasal congestion
- Postnasal drip
- Nasal polyps
- Nosebleed
- Itching
- Sneezing
- Reduced sense of smell
- Sinusitis

MOUTH AND THROAT

- Canker sores
- Dry mouth
- Excessive salivation
- Inflamed, sore lips
- Stinging tongue
- Itching roof of mouth
- Sore throat
- Hoarseness (laryngitis)
- Mucus in throat

- Dry or tickling throat
- Difficulty swallowing

NERVOUS/EMOTIONAL

- Migraine headaches*
- Hyperactivity*
- Irritability, crankiness
- Fidgeting, restlessness
- Twitching
- Numbness, tingling
- Nervousness
- Jitteriness
- Tremors
- Convulsions
- Poor coordination
- Depression, melancholy
- Drowsiness, sleepiness
- Sluggishness
- Dizziness, vertigo
- Failing memory
- Inability to concentrate
- Short attention span
- Mental confusion
- Learning disorders
- Withdrawal
- Feelings of "spaciness"
- Anxiety
- Fear or panic attacks
- Personality changes
- Behavioral problems
- Uncontrolled anger
- Emotional outbursts
- Stammering
- Dyslexia
- Crying attacks
- Insomnia
- Nightmares

- Hallucinations, delusions
- Paranoia

EARS

- Recurring ear infections*
- Fluid in ears
- Inflamed inner ear (otitis media)
- Earache
- Popping sound
- Ringing (tinnitus)
- Hypersensitivity to sound
- Itching
- Excessive ear wax
- Intermittent dizziness
- Flushing, red ear lobes
- Vertigo

MISCELLANEOUS

- Anemia
- Autoimmune disorders
- Fibrocystic breast disease
- Uterine fibroids

ALMOST ANY FOOD

Almost any food can cause adverse reactions, depending on one's unique susceptibility to it. Some people react to food additives, such as monosodium glutamate (MSG), sulphiting agents, benzoate preservatives, and tartrazine food colorings. Most food sensitivities, however, are to common natural foods – including milk products, wheat, eggs, chocolate, caffeine, oranges, strawberries, peanuts, nuts, corn, potatoes, sugar, shellfish, tomatoes, pork, beef, sugar, and soy.

The following is a list of the foods and food constituents that are commonly associated with food sensitivities, including both allergies and intolerances. There is no attempt to distinguish between the two types of reaction in this list, because what one person may be allergic to another can be intolerant of (and vice versa). On a worldwide basis, dairy products and cereal grains are the two most common food sensitivities. That is why they are placed at the head of this list. The other factors, however, are not ranked in any order of predominance.

- Cow's milk.
- Lactose – milk sugar, found in all dairy products.
- Wheat.
- Gluten – a protein in wheat, rye, oats, barley, kamut, spelt.
- Eggs.
- Chocolate – contains the alkaloid, theobromine.
- Caffeine – an alkaloid in coffee, tea, and cola drinks.
- Peanuts.
- Nuts.
- Corn.
- Oranges.
- Strawberries.
- Shellfish.
- Pork.
- Fish.
- Soy.
- Nightshades – tomatoes, potatoes, peppers, paprika, cayenne, chili, eggplant, tobacco.
- Solanine – alkaloid found in potato sprouts and tomatoes.
- Sucrose – table sugar.
- Tyramine – found in aged cheeses (e.g., blue, brie, Camembert, Gouda, Roquefort), beer, broad bean pods, chicken liver, fermented sausages, pickled herring, red wine, salami, sour cream, soy sauce, yeast.
- Salicylates – found in almonds, apples, apricots, blackberries, boysenberries, cherries, cucumbers, currants, gooseberries, grapes, nectarines, oranges, peaches, plums, prunes, raisins, raspberries, strawberries, tomatoes.
- Oxalates – found in cranberries, chard, rhubarb, gooseberries, spinach, beet leaves.

- Purines –products of digestion of alcohol, sugars, fried foods, meat, liver, kidney, fish, fowl, spinach, lentils, mushrooms, peas, asparagus.
- Sulphites – preservatives used in salad bars.
- Nitrites, Nitrates – preservatives used in processed meats.
- Monosodium glutamate (MSG) – flavour enhancer.
- Tartrazine dyes – yellow food coloring.
- Benzoates – food preservatives.
- Aspartame – an artificial sweetener.
- Butylated hydroxytoluene (BHT) – a food preservative.
- Butylated hydroxyanisole (BHA) – a food preservative.

\You are a unique individual, not a statistic. The food factors that cause problems for most sensitive people may or may not affect you. You need to investigate your own body. The above list is offered simply as a starting point for your own personal research.

WHICH FOOD, WHICH SYMPTOM

For the most part, sensitivity reactions are unique to the individual experiencing them. It is the rare exception for a particular food (or ingredient) to bring on exactly the same symptoms in everyone who is susceptible to it. One of these exceptions is the sensitivity to monosodium glutamate (MSG), a flavour enhancer popular in Asia. This food additive characteristically causes chest pain, a sensation of facial pressure, headaches, burning sensations, and excessive sweating that has been dubbed "Chinese restaurant syndrome".

A partial exception to the principal of unique responses can be made for sensitivity to the nightshade family of plants (e.g.., tomatoes, potatoes, peppers, eggplant, tobacco). These foods can and do bring on a diversity of reactions in different people – anything from irritable bowel to fluid retention and high blood pressure. Their most common symptom, however, is arthritis. An estimated 70 percent of arthritics may be sensitive to nightshades. Unless they eliminate these foods from their diets completely, nothing else they do for their condition will be completely effective.

Aspartame, an artificial sweetener, is an interesting case in point. Most people who are sensitive to it experience headaches; however, dozens of other reactions have been reported. These include anxiety, blindness, blurred vision, fatigue, hearing loss, hyperactivity, insomnia, joint pain, memory loss, menstrual cramps, muscle pain, nausea, numbness of extremities, personality changes, rapid heartbeat, seizures, skin rashes, slurred speech, suicidal depression, vertigo, and weight gain. Aspartame contains about 10 percent methyl (wood) alcohol, a known poison. That makes it toxic to just about everyone, depending on the amount consumed. Some people apparently have a higher tolerance to aspartame than others and do not develop symptoms from reasonable levels of intake. In those with a low tolerance, a wide diversity of reactions is possible – depending on each person's unique susceptibility.

Recurrent ear infections in children are most commonly caused by a sensitivity to milk products. Excess mucus produced by the sensitivity makes the adenoids swell and plugs the Eustachian tubes, allowing bacteria to grow in the middle ear (*otitis media*).

With the exception of the above handful of examples, there is usually only a very loose correlation between the symptom and the food(s) causing it. The following is a rough guide to *some* symptoms that have frequently been related to certain foods. It is by no means complete. Some of the conditions listed may have other possible causes not related to food sensitivities. Most of the foods will cause symptoms other than those listed. This partial list may be helpful as a starting point for investigating possible sensitivities. It could be misleading if routinely applied to any particular individual. Almost any food can cause almost any symptom in a susceptible person.

Abdominal pain - lactose, gluten.
Anaphylaxis - egg, peanuts, milk, fish.
Arthritis - wheat, corn, milk, nitrates, nightshades (potatoes, tomatoes, eggplant, peppers, cayenne, chili, tobacco).
Bed-wetting - milk, chocolate, citrus juices, tomatoes, pineapple, peaches.
Asthma - egg, nuts, fish, chocolate, gluten, tartrazine, benzoates, sulphites.
Bowel, irritable - lactose, milk, gluten, wheat, corn, tea, citrus fruit, chicken, egg, benzoates, nitrites
Canker sores - milk, cheese, wheat, tomato, vinegar, lemon, pineapple, mustard, gluten.
Colds, frequent - dairy products, sugar, wheat, eggs.
Colitis, ulcerative - lactose, milk, gluten.
Crohn's disease - gluten, lactose, soya, egg, milk, tomatoes, nuts.

Dermatitis - gluten, milk, egg.

Ear infections - milk products.

Eczema - egg, milk, wheat, gluten, citrus fruit, tomatoes.

Edema - wheat, cow's milk, eggs, corn, coffee, tea, alcohol, yeast, citrus fruit, sugar, tomatoes.

Epilepsy - gluten, milk, peanuts, aspartame, salicylates.

Gallbladder - egg, pork, onion, poultry, milk, coffee, citrus fruit, corn, beans, nuts.

Gastrointestinal - milk, lactose, gluten, sucrose, eggs, nuts, seafood, soya.

Gout - purines.

Heartbeat, irregular - milk, eggs.

Hives - gluten, milk, eggs, peanuts, fish, benzoates, tartrazine, monosodium glutamate, sulphites.

Hyperactivity - sucrose, milk, salicylates, BHT, BHA, artificial colors or flavors.

Hypertension - caffeine, alcohol, tomatoes.

Migraines - cheese, tomatoes, chocolate, coffee, tea, milk, egg, orange, wheat, red wine, aspartame, tartrazine, tyramines, benzoates, nitrates, nitrites.

Multiple sclerosis - milk, coffee, chocolate, colas.

Psoriasis - gluten.

Tinnitus - salicylates

Vasculitis - wine, vinegar.

As a youngster, I witnessed an uncle suffering from painful bouts of iritis (inflammation of the iris of the eye), for which painkillers were of little help. I also noticed that he addictively snacked on redskin peanuts, from dishes beside his favorite chair and at other strategic locations. When I first learned about allergic addiction, some 25 years later, this uncle immediately popped into mind.

FOOD FAMILIES

Whenever a particular food is found to which one is sensitive, it is wise to consider the botanical or zoological family from which it comes. If you are allergic or intolerant to one food in a family, you may also be sensitive to some or all of the others as well. It is not necessarily so, however.

Sometimes only one food in the family is the culprit. Individual testing is required to know for sure.

The following list summarizes foods, spices and herbs by family. If sensitive to one in a family, treat the others as suspect until demonstrated otherwise.

Algae	chlorella, spirulina.
Apple	apple, cider, cider vinegar, pectin.
Banana	banana, plantain, psyllium.
Beech	beech, chestnut, oak.
Birch	birch, filbert, hazelnut.
Borage	borage, comfrey, lungwort.
Buckthorn	buckthorn, cascara sagrada, jujube.
Buckwheat	buckwheat, rhubarb, sorrel (garden).
Buttercup	aconite, buttercup, celandine, hepatica.
Cashew	cashew, mango, pistachio.
Citrus	angostura bitters, citric acid, grapefruit, kumquat, lemon, lime, orange, tangelo, tangerine.
Cola Nut	chocolate, cocoa, cola.
Composite	arnica, blessed thistle, boneset, burdock, camomile, chicory, chrysanthemum, dandelion, elecampagne, endive, escarole, globe artichoke, Jerusalem artichoke, lettuce, romaine, oyster plant, safflower, salsify, sunflower seed, tarragon, wormwood, yarrow.
Ebony	date plum, persimmon.
Fungi	antibiotics, moldy cheese, mushroom, yeasts.
Gentian	centaury, gentian.
Ginger	cardamom, ginger, turmeric.
Gooseberry	currant, gooseberry.
Goosefoot	beet, lamb's quarters, quinoa, spinach, sugar beet, Swiss chard, thistle.
Gourd	acorn squash, cantaloupe, cucumber, honeydew melon, pumpkin, pumpkin seed, vegetable marrow, watermelon, zucchini.

Grape	brandy, champagne, cognac, cream of tartar, grape, raisin, vermouth, wine, wine vinegar.
Grass	bamboo shoots, barley, beer, bran, cane sugar, citronella, corn, dextrose, flour, glucose, grass, lemon grass, liqueurs, malt, millet, molasses, oats, pumpernickel, rice, rum, rye, sorghum, wheat, wheat germ, whiskey, wild rice.
Heather	bearberry, blueberry, cranberry, heather, huckleberry, uva ursi, wintergreen.
Honey	bee nectar, beeswax, honey, propolis, royal jelly.
Honeysuckle	elderberry, honeysuckle.
Laurel	avocado, bay leaf, camphor, cinnamon, laurel, sassafras.
Legume	acacia, alfalfa, arabic bean, black-eyed pea, broad bean, carob, cassia, chick pea, clover, fenugreek, field pea, garbanzo, green bean, green pea, gum tragacanth, jicima, kidney bean, kudzu, lentil, licorice, lima bean, locust bean, lucerne, mung bean, navy bean, peanut, pinto bean, senna, snow peas, soy bean, St. John's bread, string bean, tamarind, tonka bean, wax bean.
Lily	adder's tongue, aloe vera, asparagus, chives, garlic, leek, onion, sarsaparilla, shallot, Solomon's seal.
Linseed	flax, linseed.
Mallow	cottonseed, gumbo, hibiscus, okra.
Maple	elder, maple, maple sugar.
Mint	balm, basil, bergamot, betony, catnip, horehound, hyssop, lavender, marjoram, menthol, mint, oregano, pennyroyal, peppermint, rosemary, sage, savory, spearmint, thyme.
Morning glory	sweet potato, yam.
Mulberry	breadfruit, fig, hops, marijuana, mulberry.
Mushroom	mushroom, truffle.

Mustard	broccoli, Brussels sprouts, cabbage, cauliflower, Chinese cabbage, collards, horseradish, kale, kohlrabi, mustard, radish, rutabaga, sauerkraut, turnip, watercress.
Myrtle	allspice, bayberry, clove, eucalyptus, guava, myrtle, rose apple.
Nettle	hashish, marijuana, nettle, oregano, verbena.
Nightshade	banana pepper, bell pepper, belladonna, capsicum, cayenne, chili pepper, curry, eggplant, paprika, peppers, pimento, potato, tabasco, tobacco, tomato.
Nutmeg	mace, nutmeg.
Orchid	gum guaiacum, vanilla (true).
Palm	coconut, date, sago.
Papaw	papain, papaw, papaya, passion fruit.
Parsley	angelica, anise, asafetida, caraway, carrot, celery, chervil, cilantro, coriander, cumin, dill, fennel, gotu kola, lovage, parsley, pasnip, sweet cicely.
Pine	gin, juniper, pine, pinon.
Plum	almond, apricot, cherry, nectarine, peach, plum, prune, wild cherry.
Poppy	heroin, morphine, opium, poppy.
Purslane	New Zealand spinach, purslane.
Rose	blackberry, boysenberry, dewberry, hawthorn, loganberry, raspberry, rose hip, strawberry.
Seaweed	agar, carrageenan, dulse, hiziki, Irish moss, kelp, kombu, nori, wakame.
Tapioca	castor bean, castor oil, tapioca.
Walnut	black walnut, butternut, English walnut, hickory nut, pecan.
Yeast	baker's yeast, brewer's yeast, torula yeast.
Bass	bass, bluegill, perch, pumpkinseed, snapper, sunfish.
Cattle	beef, bison, buffalo, goat, sheep (butter, cheese, milk, ghee, yogurt).
Cod	cod, haddock, pollack, scrod, silver hake.
Crustacean	crab, crayfish, lobster, prawn, shrimp.

Deer	deer, venison, elk.
Flounder	flounder, halibut, sole.
Herring	herring, menhaden, shad.
Mackerel	bluefish, mackerel, swordfish, tuna.
Moose	moose, caribou, reindeer.
Mollusk	abalone, clam, scallop, mussel, oyster, snail, squid.
Perch	muskellunge, pickerel, pike, walleye, yellow perch.
Quail	chicken, guinea fowl, pheasant, quail, and their eggs.
Reptile	turtle, snake.
Salmon	salmon, trout
NO Family	(Unrelated to each other or to any group): arrowroot, Brazil nut, coffee, litchi nut, linden, macadamia nut, olive, pear, pepper (black and white), pineapple, pomegranate, quince, quinine, rutin, saffron, sesame, slippery elm, St. John's wort, tea.

ALLERGIC REACTIONS

Having a food allergy is like being in a state of war with a substance that the body considers to be foreign and threatening. If our immune resources are strong, we may be able to win some battles for a long while and not notice any reaction to the offending food. If we persist in eating that food, however, we may eventually lose the war. Symptoms suddenly appear, and we do not know where they came from.

An allergic reaction is an inflammation or irritation of tissues caused by an interaction between a foreign sensitizing substance (antigen) and the body's defence mechanisms. Most food allergies appear to arise when specific food antigens (protein markers) find their way past the defences of the digestive tract and into the blood (or lymph) circulation.

In immediate onset allergies, foreign proteins cause the body to produce specific IgE antibodies (immunoglobulins) that bind to the invading antigens. In the ensuing battle, powerful substances are released – including histamine, lysosomal enzymes, kinin, bradykinin, and singlet oxygen radicals. These are highly destructive and inflammatory agents that damage the body's own tissues, usually causing symptoms such as the following within 30 minutes or so: asthma, edema, sinus congestion, gastrointestinal reactions, hives, intestinal spasms, itchy eyes, nasal discharge, skin rashes, sneezing. The degree of allergenicity determines the degree of response. Less allergenic proteins that get into the blood may elicit antibodies but without inducing hypersensitivity reactions.

Histamine released from injured cells causes irritation and inflammation of surrounding tissues, including (a) tightening or spasms of the muscles, (b) dilation of blood vessels and resultant fluid leakage, (c) excess secretions of mucus, and (d) depression. Lysosomal enzymes digest and destroy tissue. Kinin and bradykinin produce inflammation. Singlet oxygen radicals destroy cellular membranes, accelerate the aging process, and contribute to such degenerative diseases as arthritis, atherosclerosis and cancer.

In delayed onset allergies, symptoms may not appear until from 48 to 72 or more hours after eating the allergenic food. These kinds of reactions appear to involve IgG antibodies, IgG immune complexes, IgM and IgA antibodies, and cellular (T-lymphocyte) mediated responses. This delayed type of allergic response is not detected by conventional skin prick tests.

Inflammation is a common allergic response, but exactly what is inflamed varies from person to person. If inflammation is in the skin it produces rashes – in the joints, arthritis – in the bladder, frequent urination or bladder infections. Inflammation of the bowel can produce bloating, constipation, diarrhea, gas, mucous colitis, nausea, or spastic colon. Inflammation of brain cells can produce delusion, depression, difficulty concentrating, dizziness, fatigue, hallucinations, headache, hyperactivity, learning disorders, manic behavior, mental fog, mood swings, poor memory, or seizures. Any part of the body can be affected. Different people allergic to the same food can have widely varying symptoms.

We usually think of an allergic reaction as something that happens immediately – such as anaphylactic shock from eating peanuts, asthmatic attacks from sulphites, or hives from pumpkin flavoured ice cream. These are all *acute* reactions from obvious causes. Other acute reactions include sneezing, wheezing, swelling, vomiting, cramps, fainting or headaches triggered by eating an uncommon food (e.g., strawberries, shellfish, nuts) or a common food infrequently (e.g., peanuts, chocolate, oranges).

Many allergic responses, however, are chronic, vague and not apparently related to the ingestion of any particular food. That makes them insidious and difficult to detect. Examples of chronic sensitivity reactions include persistent fatigue, general malaise, fleeting joint pains, headaches, a runny nose, mild feelings of unease, or any symptom that comes and goes for no apparent reason.

Persistence can convert an acute reaction into a chronic one. One example is a mother who insists on feeding cow's milk to her child, who continually spits it up. But Mom keeps pouring the milk into Junior, in the mistaken belief that he cannot be healthy without it. Eventually the child can keep the milk down and may even grow to like it. The acute reaction is gone, but only because it has become converted to chronic responses – such as recurrent ear infections, frequent colds, hyperactivity, bed-wetting, or tonsillitis. These the child may eventually grow out of, only to develop unexplained depression, headaches, and chronic diarrhea in later life – all ultimately related to the milk sensitivity.

Allergies are great masqueraders. They can mimic just about any ailment and can affect almost any part of the body. Some symptoms can be vague, others devastating. Each person has target organs that are more vulnerable than others. For example, an allergy to one specific food could – in different people – cause spasms in the bladder, a spastic colon, or spasms in the back and neck muscles. Sometimes the brain becomes a target organ, resulting in schizophrenia or other psychological or behavioral disturbances.

Some of the more common food offenders likely to cause allergic problems include: milk, wheat, corn, chocolate, egg, orange, peanut, potato, sugar, shellfish, tomato, pork and beef. Some people, however, can develop allergies to just about any food. In other words, take nothing for granted. Almost any symptom could be caused by almost any food – depending on each person's particular vulnerabilities.

Allergy and addiction are two sides of the same coin. Any foods that we continually crave or feel we cannot do without are usually the culprits causing untoward bodily responses. The adverse effects of offending foods can be dulled to some extent by eating more of the same thing – hence the expression, "more of the hair of the dog that bit you." Many people who have food sensitivities experience a low blood sugar attack (hypoglycemia) within hours of eating the foods to which they are sensitive. When blood sugar falls, you naturally crave more of the substance that made you feel good (i.e., to bring the blood sugar back up). It is the same yo-yo effect experienced by the alcoholic who has to drink in order to avoid a hangover (an allergic withdrawal reaction.) It is also the same compulsion experienced by smokers, the vast majority of whom are allergic to tobacco. It is possible to become just as addicted to a food as it is to alcohol or cigarettes.

Chocolate in some people, for example, produces nervousness and emotional upset. Some so affected have learned that these feelings can be ameliorated (at least for a short time) by eating more chocolate. This pattern can lead to an addictive pattern whereby the more one eats of a particular food, the more she or he feels compelled to eat. Continually binging on one specific food is invariably caused by a hidden allergy to it.

When any addictive substance is withheld, withdrawal symptoms are likely to develop. When the addictive substance is then consumed, the withdrawal symptoms subside and normal functioning can be resumed. Food-sensitive people are often unaware of their compulsions, yet include in their diet a daily dose of the addictive food or beverage. Through repeated stimulation they delay the withdrawal phase, thus masking the allergy. Repeated overstimulation, however, eventually leads to exhaustion. Sooner or later the adaptive mechanism breaks down and is no longer able to postpone or prevent the withdrawal state.

GALLBLADDER SENSITIVITY

Some people acquire a low tolerance to most forms of dietary fat. Eggs, pork, fried and other fatty and greasy foods cause nausea, headaches, bloating or abdominal distress. Such reactions are usually caused by insufficient bile, owing to liver/gallbladder weakness or gallstones. Certain other foods may also aggravate a gallbladder condition, such as onions, garlic, cabbage, Brussels sprouts, radishes, or cucumbers.

There is evidence that food allergies may cause gallbladder attacks in some people. Allergy-causing foods may cause swelling of the bile duct, resulting in restricted bile flow from the gallbladder. Almost any food could theoretically produce this effect in a sensitive person. Some of the possible culprits linked to gallbladder attacks include milk, coffee, citrus fruit, corn, beans, and nuts.

People with a gallbladder sensitivity can usually digest butter without difficulty. This is because the fat in butter is pre-emulsified and does not require bile for its digestion. It is completely broken down by gastric lipase in the stomach. Such is nature's way to ensure that infant mammals get all the essential fatty acids that their mother's milk provide before their own digestive system is ready to handle fats from other sources.

HIGH BLOOD PRESSURE

Hypertension is a condition in which a person has higher blood pressure (BP) than is deemed normal. Most cases of high blood pressure are caused by hidden food allergies. There is a quick way to find out for sure. For four days, drink only purified water. Consume no solid or liquid food of any kind. If hidden food allergies are involved, at the end of the four days, blood pressure will be normal. By cutting out all foods one automatically eliminates the ones causing the problem. To find out which foods are the culprits, add back one food at a time and take blood pressure readings. If no elevation in blood pressure is experienced within three hours of eating a particular food, eat another, and so on until one is found that does elevate blood pressure. Then, wait until blood pressure returns to normal before testing another food (which could be up to 12 hours). [*Caution: it is unwise for anyone with insulin-dependent diabetes to fast.*]

A less extreme way to find the allergenic foods is to measure blood pressure first thing upon arising in the morning, before any food or beverage is consumed. After breakfast take another blood pressure reading. Throughout the day, take a BP reading before and after every food or beverage that is consumed. If the upper BP reading increases by more than 14 mm. Hg over the baseline morning measurement, it is due to something eaten between arising and the high reading. Backtrack using the process of elimination to isolate the culprit(s). Frequent readings will reveal the pattern. Almost any food can cause high blood pressure; however, the most common offenders include caffeine (coffee, tea, colas), and the nightshades (tomatoes, peppers, potatoes, paprika, eggplant, cayenne, chili, tobacco). Hypertension that is caused by hidden food allergies does not respond to any treatment except the elimination of the offending foods.

A graduate student of mine called one day to ask what to do for a 23-year old client of hers who had blood pressure of 220 over 100. I suggested that if she put him on a total fast (water only) for four days, his blood pressure would return to normal. Three days later she called to say that not only was his blood pressure normal, but that she had found him to be allergic to tomatoes and had been putting ketchup on everything.

It is the first time that a substance is consumed on a particular day that is most significant. Once blood pressure has been elevated, it may stay at that higher level for the rest of the day, or for several days. Therefore, the *first* time you notice that a particular food or beverage causes an apparent rise in blood pressure eliminate it *totally* from your diet and stop testing for the rest of the day and for the next five days. It could take that long for residual reactions to this food/beverage to clear from your body. At the end of five days, resume blood pressure testing again.

Relating elevated blood pressure to specific foods can be an eye-opener for many people, especially doctors. Many cases of hypertension are termed "essential," meaning "without apparent cause." Most of the conditions for which western medicine has not yet found a cause may in time be found to involve hidden food sensitivities.

Blood pressure testing for food sensitivities will not work for anyone whose blood pressure is unaffected by them, nor will it necessarily find all sensitivities. A person could experience hypertension from some foods and still be allergic or intolerant to others that do not affect his or her blood pressure.

MIGRAINE HEADACHES

A migraine headache is one that affects one half of the head and may be accompanied by disordered vision and gastrointestinal disturbances. There may also be sharp stabbing pains in the temple region. Migraines are usually caused by hidden food allergies. Almost any food could be involved, and the most common offenders include alcoholic beverages (especially red wine), aspartame, caffeine, cheese, chocolate, milk, nitrates and nitrites, and tyramine (found in aged cheeses, fermented sausages, and sour cream). Sometimes migraine headaches can be caused or aggravated by hypoglycemia.

IRRITABLE BOWEL

Both the small and large intestines are involved in this syndrome of impaired intestinal motility. Symptoms include cramping, usually in the lower abdomen, and constipation alternating with diarrhea. The pain is usually relieved by the passage of either small-diameter stools of varying consistency or gas and mucus. Symptoms may be chronic or occur at intervals, and are often triggered by anxiety-producing periods of stress.

Irritable bowel syndrome (IBS) is invariably caused by hidden food allergies. The colons of some people are so sensitive that they react to certain common foods as if they were poisons. The aggravating foods differ from one person to the next but may include such things as wheat, milk products, oranges and citrus fruit, caffeine (coffee, tea, colas), and/or the nightshade family (tomatoes, potatoes, eggplant, peppers, paprika, cayenne, chili, tobacco).

The typical irritable bowel flares up during periods of stress because of the threshold effect on weak adrenal glands. Food allergies create a continual low-grade form of stress that is always there. Working creates stress. So do family and social situations. During times of low stress, the adrenal glands may be able to cope with allergy induced stress without displaying any symptoms. Stresses pile up, however. On high stress days the adrenals become overworked and cannot cope with the irritating foods. It is as if each person has a threshold of stress beyond which allergic symptoms are experienced but below which they are not. Strengthening the adrenal glands nutritionally can raise this threshold considerably.

COLITIS

Colitis is inflammation of the colon. In severe cases the colon can become ulcerated. Symptoms include the passage of offensive watery stools with mucus and pus, abdominal pain or tenderness, and intermittent or irregular fever.

Colitis is invariably caused by hidden food allergies. The colons of some people are so sensitive that they react to certain common foods as if they were poisons. The aggravating foods differ from one person to the next but may include such things as wheat, milk products, oranges and citrus fruit, caffeine (coffee, tea, colas), and/or the nightshade family (tomatoes, potatoes, eggplant, peppers, paprika, cayenne, chilli, tobacco). Tracking down and eliminating the offending foods relieves this condition. Total relief does not come, however, until every molecule of the culprits are eliminated from the diet.

TRACKING DOWN THE CULPRITS

If every offending food produced an immediate and obvious reaction, then the road back to health would be short and quick. Just stop eating those foods that don't agree with you. The problem is that most people do not know which foods are bothering them. Most reactions are chronic and often have no apparent relation to specific foods or even to diet itself. This is particularly true if the foods are eaten frequently and the symptoms are present most of the time.

Food sensitivities tend to occur in clusters. Rarely does anyone have just one. Furthermore, reactions to particular foods are complex. Sometimes people build a tolerance to small amounts of a particular food offender and have no apparent reaction to it until their daily intake of it exceeds a particular level. Sometimes cooking denatures allergenic proteins enough so that they do not provoke immune responses; a person may react to a particular food eaten raw but not cooked. In some cases, reactions to foods may be immediate; in others they may take hours or even days. The more frequently an inciting food is eaten, the less immediate its symptoms tend to be.

Traditional skin prick tests for allergies are perhaps only about 20 percent reliable when it comes to foods. A substance may have no reaction on the skin and yet deliver devastating consequences if eaten. Something may irritate the skin but be neutralized by digestive juices when eaten.

Sublingual testing for food allergies is more reliable than skin testing, but it is not always conclusive. This kind of test involves fasting a person for at least 14 hours and then placing drops of concentrated food extracts under the tongue to see what responses the body may have to them within the next 10 minutes or so. This form of testing can identify immediate reactions to foods but not those that are delayed. Also, it is possible that a reaction during the test could be caused by something eaten the previous day. Sublingual testing can sometimes be very harsh if the immune responses are drastic ones, such as anaphylactic shock or schizophrenic episodes. Also, sublingual tests can find only allergies, not intolerances.

There are safer tests that can be done by a nutritional practitioner who specializes in food sensitivities. Such tests include electroacupressure measuring devices such as Interro testing or EAV (electroacupuncture according to Voll), and various forms of the applied kinesiologies. This form of testing relies on detecting subtle changes in energy flow in acupressure meridians (or in muscle strength) in response to specific foods. Energy testing is affected by subjective considerations, however. Its results can be influenced by the expectations or state of mind of either the tester or the subject. In the hands of an expert who understands and knows how to eliminate the subjective element, however, energy testing methods have the potential to be very reliable and thorough. Many foods can be tested at a single sitting, without eating them and without provoking untoward responses. If properly designed, energy testing can also identify both allergies and intolerances

There is also much you can do on your own to track down dietary culprits, simply by looking for subtle clues. Suspect first those foods that you crave or feel that you cannot do without it (the allergy-addiction syndrome). Eating a problem food may cause a subtle "lift" (because of a rush of adrenal hormones) followed by a less subtle "letdown" or withdrawal. The allergic person, therefore, intuitively learns to avoid the letdown by consuming the same food (or beverage) frequently. This is exactly the same mechanism that is at work in alcoholics. Ask yourself the following hypothetical question and give the first answer to it that pops into your head: "If I were about to be marooned on a deserted island and could take only one food with me, what would it be?" Your spontaneous, automatic response to this question will very likely be a food to which you are sensitive.

Another version of this self-test is to list your five favorite foods and beverages. Look for common themes. Bread, cakes, cookies, macaroni, pasta, and pastries are all forms of wheat. Cheese, ice cream, milk, pizza and yogurt are all dairy products.

Hippocrates reported in his writings that if a food was avoided for at least four days, a re-exposure to that food could create a pronounced reaction in certain people. Modern experience reaffirms this ancient observation. Once you suspect a food, eliminate all forms of it from your diet totally for four days. Then, on the fifth day, have a serving of that food by itself. If you are sensitive to it, you will almost certainly have some noticeable reaction to it within two hours of this test meal. That is because during the abstinence your body cleared itself of all residues of it. Eating this food on the fifth day was like eating it for the first time. It is a way of converting a chronic response into an acute one by shocking your body into responding. If you suspect multiple foods, then you need to eliminate all of them at the same time. Then, add back one of the eliminated foods every five days.

Experiment with your diet. Take nothing for granted. Pay more attention to your body. If you happen to notice that you feel worse when you eat a particular food and better when you do not, then don't eat it. Eliminate it completely. No matter how important a food you (or others)

think it may be, you can always find healthy substitutes. There is no food that is indispensable.

Do not take your vitamins and food supplements for granted either. Include them as suspects in your testing program. It is impossible to manufacture tablets without excipients to shape them. Some of these fillers may include lactose, sucrose, corn, wheat, gluten, soy, yeast, colorings and preservatives. Every chewable tablet contains sugar in some form (e.g., fructose, sucrose, glucose); there is no way to make vitamins and minerals palatable without it. Look for supplements that are as hypoallergenic as possible.

Sometimes active ingredients may also be a problem for sensitive people. Allergy to vitamins, minerals and amino acids *per se* is quite rare, almost non-existent. Some people, however, may be sensitive to the source of those vitamins and minerals. For example, a vitamin C that is only 90 percent pure and derived from corn starch may trigger reactions in those who are sensitive to corn. The same holds true for B-vitamins that are derived from yeast. That is why manufacturers of hypoallergenic formulas use ingredients that are as pure as possible.

Allergy to certain herbs, on the other hand, is fairly common among those who have low immune function. In that respect an herb is just like a natural food. Almost any herb or spice can cause almost any symptom.

ELIMINATION DIETS

An elimination diet is one of the most direct ways to discover hidden food sensitivities. All possible suspect foods must be eliminated from the diet. Only those foods that are least likely to cause symptoms are to be eaten. A minimum of five days (and preferably 10 to 14 days) on this hypoallergenic diet is required to allow the gastrointestinal tract and bloodstream to clear themselves from the residues of all sensitizing foods. At the end of that time, test foods are added back to the diet at the rate of one new food every three days (because some delayed reactions to foods may take up to 72 hours.)

Add foods back in the following way: For breakfast, have a significant helping of the test food. If there is no reaction, then have a little more of it with lunch. If there is still no reaction to the last food added back, keep it in the diet and test another food three days later. Whenever a reaction occurs to a food just added, make that food a prime suspect and keep it out of the diet from that day on. (Reactions to reintroduced foods tend to be more pronounced or recognizable than before the elimination diet began.) No new food is to be tested until the reaction from the last one has completely cleared. Eat only the foods you have determined are safe until this reaction is over.

The most extreme elimination diet involves starting with a five-day water-only fast (and adding only the one test food every three days). A slightly less extreme version starts with a base diet consisting of only two hypoallergenic food sources – one for protein, the other for carbohydrate. These could be provided by, say, lamb and pears – or if a more elemental approach is desired, by hydrolyzed protein supplements. Anyone embarking on such a limited diet needs to be in reasonably good health. This is too harsh an approach for someone who is malnourished.

A gentler application of this form of diagnostic dieting involves starting by eliminating all of those foods that you (a) eat four or more days per week, (b) crave or feel you cannot do without, (c) suspect make you feel bad, and (d) find give you a lift or quick energy boost. These are the foods most likely to be causing sensitivity reactions. For extra assurance, you may wish also to exclude those foods best known for their allergic potential to other people in general (e.g., milk products, wheat, eggs, chocolate, coffee, tea, corn, oranges, tomatoes, peanuts, shellfish, strawberries, pork, table sugar, soy/tofu, yeast). An elimination diet along these lines is far easier to follow than starting with a total fast and will provide a wide enough variety of foods to ensure nutritional adequacy. To be done correctly, you must restrict yourself to only those foods whose exact composition you know. Hidden ingredients in medications, food supplements and toothpaste may be sources of eliminated foods that could reduce the diagnostic value of the test diet.

On a statistical basis, most sensitivities are to foods that have historically been introduced to the human diet since the advent of agriculture (e.g., grains, dairy products, processed foods). For that reason, some people prefer to start the first phase of their elimination diets by consuming only foods as close as possible to those eaten by our stone age (paleolithic) ancestors. Such a diet includes fish, fowl, meat, eggs, fruits, seeds, nuts, greens, root vegetables, and herbal teas. It excludes *all* grains (including cereals and baked goods), *all* milk products (including cheeses and yogurt), and *all* of the following: table sugar, alcoholic beverages, margarine, artificial food additives (including colorings, flavourings and preservatives).

Sometimes very few foods need to be eliminated. Since eliminating only suspicious foods is the easiest elimination diet to follow, it is the one that ought to be tried first. If it does not go far enough or if symptoms fail to improve, a more thorough elimination can be tried later.

Ideally, the foods permitted during all phases of an elimination diet should be as whole and unadulterated as possible. Organic produce and chemical- and hormone-free meats and poultry are the foods of choice. Consuming fast foods, confections, processed foods, caffeine, alcohol and additive-laden foods or beverages during the testing period only introduces extraneous variables that may distort results. Before condemning a particular food, you want to be sure that any apparent reaction to it was actually caused by the food itself and not by some other agent added to it.

KEEPING A FOOD DIARY

During any time period of testing for food sensitivities (by whatever means), a food diary is a definite asset. On one side of the page record the specific food(s) eaten, the approximate quantity and at what exact time. On the other side record any change in signs and symptoms and the time at which it was experienced. Reactions can be rated on a scale for purposes of comparison. Pay particular attention to the presence or absence of (a) bodily symptoms as fatigue, pain, swelling, itching, diarrhea, bloating, (b) emotional symptoms as mood swings, depression, anxiety, irritability, anger, fear, and (c) mental symptoms such as dull or slow thinking, cloudy or foggy thinking.

Look for patterns. Notice if a particular reaction occurs, say, three hours after every time a specific food (or food combination) is eaten. Notice if symptoms get better or worse the longer you go without eating anything at all. Feeling better while fasting is a common response for those who have hidden food sensitivities. Feeling irritable if late for a meal suggests hypoglycemia.

A PULSE TEST

Another detection method is to take regular measurements of the pulse wherever it can be felt easily – at the wrist, ankle, neck or temple. Pulse patterns are as unique as fingerprints and can be affected by food allergies.

The number of heartbeats must be counted for a whole minute. (Counting for fifteen seconds and multiplying by four, the way it is done in the hospital, is not accurate enough for the purpose of this test.)

First thing in the morning, while still lying in bed, take a pulse measurement. Unless you are allergic to some of your bedding or something else in the room, that will probably be your baseline resting pulse rate. Throughout the day continue taking pulse readings, at rest, while you are in a sitting position. Ideally these should be taken (a) immediately before eating a meal, (b) three times after each meal at one half hour intervals, and (c) immediately before retiring. Record each pulse reading taken in this way for three days while following your usual diet. Record also all the foods you ate at each meal. At the end of the three days calculate your average minimum and average maximum pulses, and the range between the two. If this range is more than 16 beats per minute, the chances are very good that you are allergic to something in your daily diet.

On the fourth day, immediately after rising, begin experimenting by eating a *small amount* of a different single food (mono-meal) once every hour. Record your pulse just before, 30 minutes after, and 60 minutes after each feeding. Do not test any food to which you already know you are sensitive. If any food causes your pulse to rise, you need to wait until it returns to normal before testing the next food.

If a particular meal causes your pulse to increase significantly (at least 12 beats per minute above your overall average pulse or six above your average daily maximum) then there was something you just ate to which you are allergic. Some foods may cause an increase of 20 to 40 beats per minute within 10 minutes after eating them. (Note: This technique does not catch all sensitivities, however. It is a one-sided test. You could still be allergic or sensitive to something that does not affect your pulse.)

POSTURAL PULSE TEST

Postural orthostatic tachycardia syndrome (POTS) is a disorder of the autonomic nervous system that is either caused or aggravated by hidden food allergies. The autonomic nervous system controls many automatic functions of the body, including heart rate, blood pressure, digestion, and temperature. Many people with POTS have connective tissue disorders, high or low intracranial pressure, high levels of inflammation, and extreme fatigue. Some may have related conditions, such as fibromyalgia, chronic fatigue syndrome, myalgic encephalomyelitis, Ehlers-Danlos syndrome, or mast cell activation syndrome (MCAS).

"Postural orthostatic tachycardia" literally means that heartbeat becomes abnormally rapid when moving from a prone to a standing position. In order to find out if you are affected by this syndrome, you will need to take your pulse with a wrist heart rate monitor. (1) Lie down with your eyes closed in complete silence, with no one else in the room and no distractions of any kind. (2) At the end of 10 minutes in this prone position, notice your heart rate on your wrist monitor, then stand up, again with eyes closed and in total silence. (3) After 10 minutes in the standing position, notice your pulse rate. (4) Continue standing in silence with eyes closed for another 10 minutes, then notice your heart rate.

If at the end of either 10 or 20 minutes standing your pulse rate is over 25 beats per minute higher than it was lying down, this is confirmation of POTS. As an example, if your heart rate after 10 minutes of lying down was 90 bpm, then a pulse rate of 116 or higher when standing is indicative of POTS.

SENSITIVITIES IN CHILDREN

Food allergies are often influenced (but not determined) by heredity. Allergic parents tend to have allergic children. It is not the allergy to specific substances that is inherited but rather the metabolic weaknesses that makes one susceptible to allergies in general.

There is a more direct genetic link in the case of intolerances. The inability to produce a particular digestive enzyme may, in some cases, be encoded into one's DNA. Since the child's DNA is a synthesis of that from both its parents, such an enzyme deficiency can be passed on directly. If, for example, one parent is gluten intolerant, there is a good chance that one or more children will also be.

Hereditary influences may set a potential upper limit to the health that one can achieve in his or her lifetime. Regardless of what that theoretical limit for each person may be, however, very few individuals actually achieve it. Many people indulge in counterproductive dietary habits that prevent them from realizing their full potential. Most people, regardless of their heredity, can become healthier by being responsive to their bodies' nutritional cries for help.

A few genetically rare individuals with strong constitutions may smoke, drink, eat anything they like and still be active into their advanced years. One who has inherited allergic tendencies or intolerances, however, is not so well-blessed and must pay particular attention to diet in order to maintain day-to-day health and prevent degenerative diseases.

It is a sad truth that many well-meaning parents sabotage their children's nutritional development in its early stages. The infant's body was designed to thrive on its mother's milk until it is able to feed itself. The longer babies are breastfed, the less likely they are to develop food sensitivities. Human breast milk appears to protect against (and cow's milk formulas promote) the development of specific allergies.

Breast milk is the ideal food for infants. When a breastfed baby develops allergic reactions, it is more than likely in response to something the mother has been eating rather than to the breast milk itself. Diaper and skin rashes, for example, have been observed to clear up when the lactating mother stopped drinking cow's milk and eating cheese.

The two most common classes of food that westerners give their babies before their digestive systems can handle them are cereal grains (especially wheat) and cow's milk. Sensitivities to wheat and dairy products are also two of the most frequent experienced by adults. What we feed our children now can affect them for life.

Infants do not produce amylase (starch-splitting) enzymes at birth and are unable to do so for quite some time. Salivary amylase is not usually present in any appreciable quantity until about six months of age. Pancreatic amylase is not produced in adequate amounts until the molar teeth are developed – which may not be until 28 to 36 months. For these reasons, cereals, breads, crackers, cookies and other starchy foods should not be given to infants. Unfortunately, cereal is usually the first food recommended by pediatricians and dietitians.

The earlier a baby is exposed to potential allergens (allergy-provoking substances), the more likely it is to develop hypersensitivity reactions. It takes from six to nine months for the intestinal mucosal barrier to develop its proper selective permeability. Residues from inappropriate foods introduced before that time may enter the bloodstream and provoke immune responses.

The following guidelines for feeding infants help to reduce both the incidence and severity of food sensitivities that they are likely to acquire. (1) Nurse infants for as long as possible, ideally until their teeth start to bite the nipple. That's the way other mammals know when to stop suckling their young. (2) No solid foods of any kind for at least six months and preferably for one year. (3) First solid foods should be pureed meats, fruits, green leafy vegetables. (4) No cereals or starchy foods until the baby has the molars to grind them.

For infants born into allergic families, more stringent guidelines are appropriate. These babies deserve to be breastfed exclusively for at least one year. During that time the mother should practise a rotational diet in which she does not eat the same food more often than once every four or five days. Traces of whatever the mother eats may find its way into her breast milk. Having her rotate her foods will prevent her baby from being exposed to any one substance long enough or consistently enough to present a serious threat to its immune system.

WHAT IS LEFT TO EAT

The foods most likely to trigger sensitivity reactions are those eaten most frequently. The elimination of these foods, therefore, is cause for immediate concern. With what does one replace them? Dietary habits tend to be heavily ingrained and difficult to change.

Those foods to which most people are least likely to be sensitive (statistically speaking) include the following: arrowroot, artichoke, bananas, blueberries, broccoli, buffalo/bison, cranberry, deer, elk, figs, flaxseed, gelatin, lamb, macadamia nuts, moose, pears, pineapple, pistachio nuts, pumpkin, rabbit, spinach, summer squash, sweet potato, Swiss chard, tapioca, turkey, turnip, winter squash – i.e., the ones that most westerners do not eat regularly. Consider foods from this list as a starting point in planning elimination or rotational diets that you subsequently modify in light of your own experience.

If the number of foods you need to eliminate at first seems formidable, expand your perspective. There are easily over 200 foods to which you have everyday access. If you are sensitive to, say, 40 of these foods, you can still safely consume the other 80 percent. The world is far more abundant than it might seem at first glance. We are creatures of habit. We have allowed our diets to centre around a handful of foods that we consider staples. Food allergies and intolerances, however, are telling us that we need to change those habits. Consider them an opportunity to create a higher level of health you have not known before. All it takes is imagination and persistence.

Your local natural foods store can be an excellent resource for substitute foods and recipe books.

AVOIDANCE IS NOT CURE

If you want relief from food sensitivities, you must identify and eliminate the offending foods. Doing so will enable your body to recover from those conditions directly caused by those sensitivities. If you do not do this, then nothing else you do in terms of food or supplement choices will bring complete results. The causative factors will still be at work.

"A little bit won't hurt" is bad advice when it comes to food sensitivities. A little bit of a poison is still a poison. Your body could react to even one molecule of a food to which you are sensitive. To see how much of such food you can get away with would be like trying to find out how much arsenic you could safely consume each day. Total results demand a total effort.

Eliminating offending foods from the diet will begin to alleviate associated symptoms after the bloodstream has cleared itself of antibody/ antigen complexes and after the intestinal tract has cleared itself of any food residues. This process usually takes anywhere from three to five days of total avoidance of all the sensitive foods.

Troublesome foods are not always easy to identify. Some common foods (e.g., wheat, corn, soy, lactose) are hidden components in many processed foods. Label checking of ingredients is mandatory. When eating out it is often necessary to ask for assurance from the chef or cook that a particular food does not contain the factors to which you are sensitive. Restaurant personnel are quite happy to provide this information, particularly if they are led to believe that eating the wrong food could cause you to have a medical emergency in their establishment.

Avoiding the troublemakers is not a cure, however. Once you know what your particular "poisons" are, you need to be vigilant to make sure they do not creep back in – the reward for which may be better health than you could have imagined.

ROTATIONAL DIETS

The constant, monotonous intake of any food promotes the development of food allergy in sensitive people. Therefore, susceptible people need to do more than simply eliminate the offending foods. It is also recommended that they do not consume too much of any of their "safe" foods – in order not to develop sensitivities to them also. Rotational diets were developed for that purpose.

In a rotational diet, all tolerated foods are eaten no more frequently than once every four or five days. As an example, one's major protein source could be lamb one day, turkey the next, fish the next, eggs the next, then back to lamb again. This method ensures dietary diversity. The idea is that infrequent consumption of tolerated foods is not likely to induce new sensitivities. As the body becomes stronger and tolerance for eliminated foods returns, they may gradually be added back into the rotation schedule (provided that the original sensitivity to them is not permanent).

ORGANIC FOODS

Organic foods are raised without artificial fertilizers, pesticides or herbicides. In addition to being free from chemical contamination, organic foods also tend to be higher in nutrient density than their commercially raised counterparts. Consuming organic foods is thus an excellent way (a) to reduce the body's exposure to potential pollutants, and (b) to increase one's intake of vital nutrients. Both of these factors are important to those who are struggling to overcome compromised immunity, and especially to those who must follow severely restricted diets. If there are relatively few foods that one can safely consume, then one needs to derive as much nutritional benefit from them as possible.

Hundreds of extraneous chemicals find their way into our everyday foods. Many become part of the cells of the plants and cannot be washed off. Whenever reactions are noted to a particular food, it is a good idea to test both organic and commercial versions of that same food. Sometimes it is the chemical contamination of the food that is at fault; sometimes it is the food itself. Make no assumptions.

DESENSITIZATION SHOTS

Some allergists have found that by repeatedly injecting a patient with very dilute extracts of an offending food or inhalant, that person eventually no longer appears to react to that substance when exposed to it. Those who go for allergy shots, however, usually find new allergies cropping up all the time. They stop reacting to some foods only to start reacting to others.

The absence of a reaction does not necessarily mean that the allergy is gone. What desensitization shots usually do is convert acute reactions into chronic ones. The problem is still there, only buried deeper. What started out as an obvious skin or respiratory reaction, for example, may be converted to less obvious chronic fatigue or generalized malaise.

Desensitization shots do nothing to increase immunity or eliminate allergies. On the contrary; they make an already compromised immune system weaker, thus reducing the body's ability to react to substances that are toxic to it. A far better approach is to identify and support the underlying weaknesses.

ADRENAL SUPPORT

Many allergies are more pronounced under conditions of stress. One can sometimes eat a problem food on a good day and experience no adverse effects whatever. On another day, when the weather is bad, tempers are flaring, or there is stress at the office, that same food could have alarming effects. It is as if there is a threshold of resistance. All stresses (including allergic ones) pile up. If the "pile" exceeds the threshold limit, problems result. If it is a small "pile" the body may be able to handle it. Emotional stress can often be the deciding factor that pushes the stress level over the top, provoking an allergic response. When this happens, it may seem as if the emotions are the cause of the allergy rather than merely the trigger that sets them off.

Sometimes people are amazed to discover that suddenly one day, they have a problem with food sensitivities. Actually, the process may have been building up for many years. Imagine a dam with water behind it. One day it overflows, but it could have been building up to that level for 20 or 30 years.

Stress of all kinds is mediated by the adrenal glands. If these tiny glands are undernourished or overworked, they cannot do their job adequately.

Many allergies disappear when the adrenal weakness is supported with specific nutrients.

The following are nutrients specifically required for rebuilding the adrenal glands and restoring their function. An optimal range for daily supplementation is suggested beside each – ideally to be taken in divided amounts with meals:

Vitamin C	1,000 to 3,000 mg.
Pantothenic Acid	500 to 1,500 mg.
Vitamin B-12	500 to 1,000 mcg.
Adrenal concentrate	500 to 800 mg.

Any serious attempt to strengthen the adrenals must also include the elimination of concentrated and refined sugars, alcohol, caffeine and tobacco. These factors are adrenal stressors and hypoglycemic triggers, even in the absence of any specific allergy or intolerance to them.

DETOXIFICATION

Autointoxication is the pollution of our bodies from within – and it is a contributing factor to many disease processes. Every cell both takes in nutrients and discharges wastes. If waste products are not eliminated, they accumulate and prevent cells from receiving the nourishment they need. The best diet in the world and the best food supplements cannot help cells that are strangling to death in their own excretions. Toxicity causes decay and disease.

There are two important steps to every sound nutritional program: (1) detoxify, and (2) rebuild. To bypass the first is to undermine the second.

INTERNAL POLLUTION

We overload our bodies with substances that have little or no food value. Coffee, tea, tobacco smoke, drugs, artificial colorings, preservatives, artificial flavourings, agricultural chemicals, and airborne pollutants contribute to toxic overload without providing any nourishment. Alcohol, refined flours, refined sugars, soft drinks, and adulterated fats also contribute to toxic overload. These are the "empty calorie" foods that contribute no essential nutrients but require the body to work just to deal with them.

Even healthy foods can create a toxic burden if we eat too much of them – if we consume more than our bodies can digest, absorb, assimilate, and excrete. Foods to which a person is allergic or intolerant add even more toxicity, since the body cannot metabolise them properly.

The first and most important step to detoxification is to stop putting toxins into the body. Consume only healthy food (preferably organic) and only in amounts to satisfy genuine hunger.

WATER

Water provides the medium in which all biochemical reactions take place in the body. Most of our bodyweight is water. Water is needed to eliminate wastes through the kidneys and colon. Most of us do not drink enough water. It is a very healthy habit to consume from two to three litres (quarts) of purified water – preferably reverse osmosis. Make it a habit. Thirst is not a reliable indicator since by the time you feel thirsty, your body is already in the beginning stages of dehydration.

LYMPHATIC DRAINAGE

Lymph vessels are a virtual sewage system of the body. Lymph fluid is the intermediary between blood and bodily cells, in which nutrients are exchanged and waste carried off. There is more lymph in the body than blood, but it must circulate without benefit of a heart or pump. Aerobic exercise is what the lymph nodes and vessels need to massage them and keep them working efficiently.

Which kind of exercise is best? Any that causes the body to sweat for at least 22 minutes at a time, three times a week. Lymph nodes are heavily concentrated in the neck, armpit and groin – so these are the areas that need to be worked regularly. Tennis, swimming, cycling, handball, martial arts, aerobics, tai chi, brisk walking, rebounding on a mini-trampoline – all will do nicely. Do what you enjoy, so that it will be a pleasure to continue. If your body is out of shape, move into exercise very gradually. Your body thrives on activity and challenge, and keep that challenge reasonable.

ELIMINATION THROUGH THE SKIN

The skin is sometimes referred to as the "third kidney" because of its ability to release toxins through perspiration. Having a sauna twice per week is a great aid to detoxification. Infrared saunas are even better than conventional saunas for this purpose, since infrared rays have the ability to penetrate up to 3 cm. below the skin. Another method to draw toxins through the skin is to have a hot bath in which you have added one cup of sea salt and one cup of apple cider vinegar. Make the bath water as hot as you can stand and stay in it for as long as you can stand it.

LIVER CLEANSING

The liver is the master chemical factory of the body. It is the largest gland and has many important tasks to perform. The liver:

- filters virtually everything that arrives in the bloodstream.
- manufactures thousands of compounds to detoxify the body.
- readies environmental and metabolic poisons for excretion.
- metabolises glucose, glycogen, amino acids, and fatty acids.
- stores glycogen, iron, and vitamins A, D, E, K, and B-12.
- produces cholesterol, triglycerides and bile.
- breaks down worn-out red blood cells.
- acts as a blood reservoir.

The liver (among other functions) is the major organ of detoxification. It has to detoxify alcohol, environmental pollutants, toxic chemicals in food, and the toxic by-products of internal metabolism. These burdens can often overwhelm the liver. When this happens, it stores toxins in fat cells, hoping to be able to deal with them later. If the liver is kept constantly busy processing what is coming in, it never gets a chance to catch up with its "housecleaning." As toxins accumulate, they become a continual source of inflammation and deterioration.

Anything that eases our toxic burden makes the liver's job easier – including eating less, drinking more water, reducing toxic exposure, exercising more, eating more fiber, and so on. There are also a number of herbs that help the liver with its detoxification tasks. These include dandelion root, yellow dock, burdock, chickweed and barberry.

MINI-FASTING

Fasting means not eating for brief periods. In order for the liver to catch up with its housecleaning, so to speak, it sometimes needs to take a short vacation from eating.

It can be a good idea, weekly or monthly, to take a complete rest from food. Choose a 24-hour period in which you do not have to be very active. For this one day consume only two to three litres (quarts) of purified water. During this mini-fast, if you feel tired, rest. If you feel lightheaded, weak or hungry, then drink more water. You are completely in charge. If at any time you wish to end the fast, do so.

The first meal upon breaking the fast is to consist of fresh, raw vegetables or fruit – preferably organic. Gradually re-introduce heavier foods as genuine hunger indicates.

Insulin-dependent diabetics should *not* fast. To do so might cause their blood sugar levels to drop too dramatically when they take their insulin. Passive hypoglycemics may have difficulty fasting because of the blood sugar crash they characteristically experience from three to five hours after eating. Just about everyone else can safely fast for short periods, including reactive hypoglycemics, for whom blood sugar drops only in response to the ingestion of sweets, sugary foods, caffeine or alcohol.

Longer periods of fasting can be of benefit, up to a maximum of 10 days, provided that such fasts are supervised by practitioners skilled in therapeutic fasting and that select foods are gradually re-introduced from the fourth day of the fast to the tenth. Prolonged fasting is potentially dangerous as it causes the body to consume vital tissues and to shift the body into a low thyroid mode.

COLON CLEANSING

The human colon is long and convoluted. It requires lots of indigestible fiber and water to enable it to pass wastes efficiently. Fiber, the indigestible outer coating of plant cells, provides no nutrients but acts as an intestinal broom to sweep the colon clean.

When the colon becomes stagnant, toxins are reabsorbed into the bloodstream and spread throughout the body. Also, bile reacts with putrefactive bacteria to produce free radical causing chemicals in the gut (e.g., apcholic acid, 3-methyl cholanthrene).

Many people are constipated without knowing so. They assume that everything is normal as long as they have bowel movements every day. Not necessarily. Transit time is critical. Today's movement could be from a meal eaten several days ago. Eat some beets. Time how long it takes for the characteristic red stain to show up in the stools. Ideally, it should be less than 24 hours.

Oddly enough, diarrhea can be a symptom of constipation. Sometimes a colon is so badly blocked that only liquid waste can pass through. Both constipation and diarrhea disturb intestinal bacteria, so it is also a good idea to help normalize microflora by taking *Lactobacillus acidophilus* or similar probiotics.

A good way to keep the colon full of fiber is to consume about 60 percent of your food from plant sources (e.g., vegetables, whole grains, legumes, nuts, seeds, fruits). Animal products contain zero fiber.

Bran is a popular fiber supplement – but it contains phytates that bind minerals and make them unavailable to the body. Also, for those allergic or sensitive to wheat, bran can sometimes be constipating. Oat bran and rice bran are improvements over wheat bran. Finely powdered psyllium hulls, however, are the most efficient source of gently stimulating natural fiber.

Laxatives, even natural herbal ones, can be detrimental if taken on a regular basis. All laxatives work by irritating the colon, causing it to go into spasm. The more one stimulates the bowel artificially, the lazier it becomes and the more it has to depend on laxatives.

Enemas and colonic irrigation have merit during acute situations. Like laxatives, however, if used on a regular basis, they may cause the colon to become lazy and dependent upon them. Both enemas and colonics penetrate only so far into the colon, against the direction of its natural flow; and they require a skilled practitioner to administer them. Psyllium, on the other hand, can flush out the entire colon in the direction of its natural flow.

PETROLEUM DETOX

Our bodies become polluted with petrochemicals. We breathe in petroleum fumes from motor fuels, heating fuels, automobile and aircraft exhausts, smog, cleaning fluids, and paraffin candles. We expose our skins to petroleum from ointments, cosmetics, petroleum jelly, motor oils, lubricants, rust preventatives, furniture polish, and shoe polish. We consume petroleum internally from drugs, artificial food colorings, and mineral oil laxatives.

Every year in North America, acute ingestion of petroleum distillates (e.g., gasoline, kerosene, paint thinners) and halogenated hydrocarbons (e.g., carbon tetrachloride, ethylene dichloride) is responsible for poisoning over 25,000 children under the age of five. Death can come from a severe aspiration pneumonitis after accidental ingestion. Inhalation abuse of halogenated hydrocarbons by teenagers can result in sudden cardiac death.

Petroleum products are poisonous to the human body. Acute exposure to them can be fatal. Chronic, long term exposure creates a toxic overload that depresses immunity and cellular integrity – and contributes to a number of diseases, including atherosclerosis, Hodgkin's disease and various other forms of cancer. There is a very simple remedy: a homeopathic dilution of petroleum (30C) energetically stimulates the body to release its toxic burden of petroleum based products.

HEAVY METAL DETOX

Heavy metal toxicity is more common than one might imagine. Aluminum, arsenic, cadmium, lead, mercury, and nickel are heavy metals that tend to accumulate within the brain, kidneys, and immune system – where they can seriously impair normal functioning. Most heavy metals in the body are the result of industrial contaminants in the environment. Other sources can include **aluminum** from antacids and cookware; **cadmium** from fungicides, pesticides, cigarette smoke, and some plastics; **lead** from pesticide sprays, cooking utensils and soldered seams in tin cans; **mercury** from dental amalgam fillings, contaminated fish, and wood preservatives; **nickel** from nickel-plated jewellery, some metal cooking vessels, cigarette smoke, hydrogenated fats, fertilizers, and some refined foods. Workers with high exposure to heavy metals include battery makers, dentists, gasoline station attendants, printers, roofers, and solderers.

Early signs of heavy metal poisoning tend to be vague, varied, and attributed to other causes. They can include: fatigue, headache, irritability, indigestion, muscle and joint pain, tremors of the hands, anemia, pallor, constipation, abdominal cramps, dizziness, anxiety, poor coordination, skin rashes, high blood pressure, failing memory, muscular weakness, headaches, and a metallic taste in the mouth. Aluminum toxicity sometimes reveals itself as a distaste for potatoes. Cadmium toxicity may be associated with high or low blood pressure, emphysema, prostate enlargement, kidney disorders, liver disorders, and lowered immunity. Almost everyone with even mild heavy metal toxicity experiences impaired ability to think or concentrate. As toxicity increases, so do the symptoms.

A **homeopathic** formula that contains 30C concentrations of aluminum, cadmium, lead, mercury, and nickel stimulates the body energetically to reduce its toxic burden of heavy metals. An **arterial cleansing formula** that includes generous amounts of vitamin B-1 (thiamine), vitamin C, L-cysteine hydrochloride, and DL-methionine facilitates the removal of heavy metals from arteries and deep tissues.

FOOD ALONE IS NOT ENOUGH

Some people are blessed with strong constitutions. They eat whatever they like, drink, smoke, don't exercise, never take supplements – and hardly ever get sick. These genetically strong individuals, however, are becoming increasingly rare. Many are discovering that they need some form of food supplementation to keep them in optimum health.

Perhaps we could get all the nutrients we need from food alone over 100 years ago, before the dominance of "agribusiness" and processed foods. Nowadays this is becoming an increasingly naive notion. Food supplements are no substitute for eating correctly, but they can be a wonderful enhancement to it.

HYPOASCORBEMIA

Humans, apes, guinea pigs, and fruit eating bats all suffer from a genetic mutation whereby they are unable to produce ascorbate (vitamin C) in their livers the way other mammals and birds do. This means that we have to depend on external sources for this vital nutrient. What we call vitamin C is really a liver metabolite that participates in many biochemical pathways in the body.

Dr. Irwin Stone theorized that scurvy was not a dietary disturbance, but rather a potentially fatal flaw in human genetics that has been misunderstood by nutritionists. He proposed the name "hypoascorbemia" for the effects of this genetic defect and postulated that relatively large daily amounts of vitamin C are required to overcome it.

Hypoascorbemia is the reason why sailors used to develop scurvy on long voyages on which they were deprived of fruits and vegetables. Hypoascorbemia is the reason why vitamin C is beneficial to so many health conditions. According to Linus Pauling, it is also the reason why research monkeys die if they are not given 70 times the equivalent amount of C recommended for humans.

Scurvy is the name given to the most advanced stage of vitamin C deprivation, occurring just before death. Some of the early symptoms of this condition include ● tendency to bruise easily, ● hemorrhages in the eye or under the skin, ● inflamed or bleeding gums (gingivitis), ● joint pains, ● excessive hair loss, ● listlessness or fatigue, and/or ● fleeting pains in the legs. These are still fairly common symptoms among the general population. Scurvy still exists. We just don't call it by that name anymore.

Ascorbate (vitamin C) plays an active part in: (a) manufacturing collagen, the "glue" that holds bodily cells together, (b) strengthening blood vessels, (c) manufacturing hemoglobin in red blood cells, (d) secreting adrenal hormones, (e) protecting against viral and bacterial infections, (f) assimilating iron, (g) acting as an antihistamine, (h) producing interferon, an internal anti-cancer agent, and (i) manufacturing lipoprotein lipase, an enzyme that dissolves fats, including those that build up in the plaque on artery walls.

Here is a remarkable fact: animals that produce ascorbate in their livers are immune to atherosclerosis. If you wish to induce atherosclerosis in laboratory animals, you have to use monkeys or guinea pigs. Somehow, the ability to produce vitamin C internally prevents an animal's arteries from plugging up. This is probably due to at least three biochemical mechanisms: (1) vitamin C enables the body to produce lipoprotein lipase (LPL), an enzyme that dissolves fats that accumulate in arterial plaque, (2) vitamin C enables the body to produce co-enzyme Q_{10}, an antioxidant that protects arteries from the damaging effects of oxygen free radicals, and (3) vitamin C itself is a powerful antioxidant.

When all functions of vitamin C are considered, much more is needed than the puny amounts suggested by standard vitamin charts. If the human liver were capable of producing ascorbate the way other mammals do, it would probably produce a range of from 2,000 to 10,000 mg. per day (when converted for equivalent body weight). Demands for ascorbate soar during times of stress, fear, infection, or disease. It is our inability to produce vitamin C on demand that makes us vulnerable to many diseases.

It takes about 40 oranges to yield 2,000 mg. of vitamin C per day – the minimum that each human body would produce internally, if it could. Supplements make more sense, and are much more cost effective.

This is a reliable self-test to determine the minimum amount of supplementary vitamin C to maintain optimal health: On the first day, take a measured amount of vitamin C (e.g., 500 or 1,000 mg.). The second day, double this amount. The third day, triple the initial amount – and so on in ever increasing amounts. At some point, a level of intake will be reached at which a small percentage of vitamin C spills over into the urine, turning it to a bright yellow or orange color. For most adults this occurs somewhere between 1,000 mg. and 4,000 mg. daily, and it can vary from day to day. Take as much vitamin C as needed to produce brightly colored urine at least twice per day. (If you have ever seen dog or wild animal urine in the snow, it is bright yellow. Probably nature's way of ensuring the urinary tract gets enough vitamin C.)

To determine one's therapeutic level of vitamin C, continue the above self-test by increasing daily supplementation until bowel tolerance is reached. This will be the point at which the vitamin C produces either loose stools or excessive flatulence. Then, reduce that daily intake by one third. For example, if bowel tolerance is reached at a daily intake of 9,000 mg., then 6,000 mg. is the optimal therapeutic level to take during acute illness or to help overcome serious degenerative diseases.

SOIL DEPLETION

Most of North American soil is deficient in minerals – especially iodine, selenium, iron, zinc, and chromium. Modern, synthetic fertilizers deplete minerals further with each successive growing season. If the minerals are not in the soil, they will not be in our food – neither in the plants nor in the animals that eat the plants.

Plants can survive on lower mineral levels than humans can. Tasty, healthy-looking fruits and vegetables produced today now contain only a fraction of the nutrients they did in the past. The quality is not the same, however. Seventy years ago wheat was between 20 and 30 percent protein. Now we are lucky if it averages 10 percent.

Most women need, on average, about 18 mg. of iron per day for optimum health. To get this much from food alone would require eating about 3,000 calories per day – enough to maintain a body weight of some 115 Kg. (250 lb.). There are more efficient ways to get iron. One is to take a daily broad spectrum vitamin-mineral supplement containing an organic form of iron (e.g., ferrous fumarate).

LOSSES ON ROUTE

Most of us do not have the opportunity to pick and eat our fruits, vegetables, and nuts fresh from the garden. It takes a long time before food finally reaches our tables. Such are the logistics of feeding large, scattered populations.

Our produce is typically picked before it is ripe – before it has developed its full nutrient potential. It is often gassed, sprayed, shipped long distances and stored for long periods of time. Vitamin losses occur at every stage. Many of the oranges we eat, for example, have very little vitamin C left in them. That frozen juice we had from concentrate this morning may have been made from fruit picked two or three years ago. Even when we try to eat natural foods, we may not be getting everything we think we are.

FOOD PROCESSING

The more food is processed, the more nutrients it loses. Even home cooking destroys vitamins. Freezing, thawing, heating, cooking, and storing can cause oxidation, rancidity, or other destructive changes in B-vitamins, vitamin C, and fat-soluble nutrients.

The first loyalty of food companies is to their shareholders. The ideal profit-making food is one that tastes good (especially if it is addictive) and never spoils. Accordingly, commercial foods are laced with flavour enhancers and preservatives.

Most processed foods are incapable of building health. The only food that will not spoil is one that has no nutritional value left in it. If there is nothing for microbes or parasites to feed on, then there is nothing in it to nourish humans either.

Our animals are better fed than we are. We discard the valuable germ and bran of grains and put them into animal feeds. The lifeless residue we eat ourselves.

Highly processed and "junk" foods provide only carbohydrates. They are often called "empty calorie" foods. But they are actually much worse than that. "Negative foods" or "anti-nutrients" are more accurate terms. A high sugar intake causes the body to use higher amounts of B-vitamins, calcium, magnesium, zinc, and chromium. Salt tends to displace the body's potassium. Such foods take more than they give.

Artificial colorings, flavorings, and preservatives are man-made chemicals not found in nature. Some are suspected of being toxic to the human body. Some are presumed to be safe. For most, we simply do not know what the long term effects on health might be. If a substance is foreign to the human body, it cannot be utilized. It contributes nothing except extra work, because now the body has to get rid of it.

In the refining of flour, 22 nutrients are depleted. Three or four vitamins and iron are added back in small amounts, and the end product is referred to as "enriched." "Devitalized" would be a more accurate term. The more processed foods we eat, the more we need to take supplements.

STRESS MAKES EXTRA DEMANDS

The hustle-bustle western lifestyle creates nutritional stresses unknown to our ancestors. We bolt down food on-the-run. We eat at fixed times, even when not hungry. We live in homes, offices, and automobiles that are sealed off from the environment. We breathe air and drink water that becomes more polluted each year. We are bombarded with stray radiation. We don't exercise enough. We consume alcohol, tobacco, caffeine, and various medications. We go on fad or crash diets. We deprive ourselves of sleep. We do not spend enough time outdoors. Each of these factors puts extra nutritional demands on our bodies. The more of them that pile up, the greater our need for supplements.

BIOCHEMICAL INDIVIDUALITY

We all have different fingerprints, voices, and outward appearances. Internally we are just as different. Certain organs may be genetically weak or differ in size, shape, or ability from person to person. Such physical differences often result in widely differing needs for specific nutrients related to those organs.

Research suggests that some people may need from four to 40 times the amount of certain nutrients that others do. With such widely differing needs, generalizations about dietary intake are useless. Those who have unusually high requirements need to take supplements in order to achieve optimum health.

We also differ in our ability to utilize nutrients. As we age, our production of digestive juices declines. Some of us have inefficient intestinal absorption. Even if we eat the best food, we have to absorb it before it can do us any good. Sometimes we need extra nutrients to compensate for digestive weakness.

DRUGS DEPLETE NUTRIENTS

Socially acceptable drugs (e.g., alcohol, caffeine, nicotine) are drugs nonetheless. They contribute to diseases of the lungs, pancreas, liver, and gastrointestinal tract. They also interfere with our bodily utilization of many vitamins, minerals, and trace nutrients.

Pharmaceuticals pose even greater risks. They interfere with cellular biochemistry. That is how they work: by blocking metabolic pathways in the body. This action has the unfortunate consequence of preventing nutrients from being fully utilized. The most commonly used nutrient-depleting drugs are laxatives, antacids, pain-killers, antibiotics, and birth control pills.

LACK OF EXERCISE

We use our cars rather than our feet. We spend long sedentary hours in front of desks, computers, or television sets. We seldom engage in regular exercise programs. Such inactivity has nutritional consequences. It contributes to poor circulation and inadequate lymphatic drainage, thereby reducing the efficiency with which nutrients are delivered to and waste products removed from individual cells in the body.

Our bodily requirements are much the same as our paleolithic ancestors, who hunted and foraged all day. They ate far more than we do. They had to, in order to support their higher energy requirements. More food provides more calories – and also more vitamins, minerals, and trace elements. Even if we eat the best quality organic food, on 2,000 calories per day we are getting only half the nutrients that our primitive ancestors did on their 4,000 calorie diets. (And those on reducing diets may be getting only one quarter of what paleolithic humans did.)

DIETARY BALANCE

Conventional advice about nutrition is oversimplified. Merely eating from four basic food groups ignores the varying nutrient densities of different foods. Whole, natural foods tend to be concentrated sources of fiber, vitamins, and minerals when compared to their processed counterparts. The more refined foods we eat, the greater our need for supplements.

By eating a little of everything many naively assume that they will be getting everything their bodies require. It is not that simple. Most common foods are over-processed and under-vitalized. Nutrient tables are misleading. Does that cup of broccoli, for example, provide 140 mg. of vitamin C or next to none? It depends on where and when it was harvested, how rich or poor the soil was, and what has happened to it since.

Nutrient tables are misleading in their simplicity. They characteristically list only six vitamins and four minerals. No mention is made of the other 14 or so that we need.

Recommended daily intakes (RDAs, RNIs) are useless for building optimal health. They represent the least amount of a given nutrient that will prevent advanced deficiency diseases (e.g., scurvy, beri beri, rickets, goitre), plus a small margin. These numbers are generated by committees who take an average guess at what they think the average person needs for each vitamin and mineral. They totally ignore the many subclinical deficiency states that preceded the disease in question. They also ignore the widely differing needs of individuals. RNIs and RDAs may also be subject to political pressure from food processors, who do not want their low nutrient foods to look bad by comparison

There is no reliable way to know the exact quantities of nutrients that any particular food provides. Taking broad-spectrum supplements is one way to make sure that nothing is left to chance.

BUILDING SUPERIOR HEALTH

Many consider nutrition only as insurance against disease. Much more is possible. Athletes and bodybuilders continually strive to improve; they are not content with average performance. Similarly, growing numbers of people do not want average nutrition. They want the best possible. They want to feel vitally alive every day. This state can be achieved, but only if we give our bodies everything they need. Every bodily cell is manufactured from the nutrients we digest, absorb, and assimilate. It makes sense. We need to consume generous amounts of high quality nutrients if we want to build superior bodies – and that requires taking supplements.

NUTRIENTS, NOT DRUGS

Some people are reluctant to take food supplements because they associate them with drugs. The two classes of substance are worlds apart. The only thing they have in common is an outward appearance (i.e., tablet or capsule). How they behave in the body is profoundly different, in at least eight different ways:

1. **Drugs are foreign to the human body.** They do not become part of our tissues, nor do they contribute nutrients.
2. **Drugs are powerful chemical agents** that alter bodily functions by interfering with biochemical reactions and enzymatic processes.
3. **Drugs produce side effects**, many of which can be permanent. Even aspirin can cause stomach upset, internal bleeding, nausea, impaired vision, mental confusion, rashes, ringing in the ears, digestive disturbances, and death.
4. **Drugs are potentially lethal**. Misuse and overdoses can kill. (Death is the most permanent side effect of all.)
5. **Drugs deal with symptoms, not causes**. They tend to mask difficulties rather than correct them. There is no bodily condition that is caused by the deficiency of any drug. Headaches, for example, are not caused by a lack of aspirin.
6. **Drugs have to be monitored carefully** to prevent harmful overdoses and untoward side reactions.
7. **Drugs cause diseases**. In North America there is an alarming growth of those diseases termed "iatrogenic" (physician caused).
8. **Drugs cannot prevent disease**. One does not take analgesics to prevent headaches, nor chemotherapy to prevent cancer. Nutrients protect against disease by strengthening cells against invaders and by slowing down degenerative processes.

Nutrients, including dietary supplements, are quite different. There is no way that a drug can substitute for a vital nutrient.

1. **Nutrients are natural and essential.** If our intake is inadequate, we die or suffer impaired functioning.
2. **Nutrients work by supporting** biochemical and enzymatic processes.
3. **Nutrients rarely produce side effects.** Overuse of a few of them can induce temporary, reversible symptoms of overload. Because the body has built-in enzyme systems to handle nutrients, it can readily deal with excesses.
4. **Nutrients are safe.** According to poison control statistics, there has never been a single documented fatality caused by taking vitamin, mineral, or amino acid supplements.
5. **Nutrients correct conditions** caused by their lack.
6. **Nutrients are readily self-administered.**
7. **Nutrients prevent diseases.**
8. **Nutrients can achieve superior wellness** and not merely the absence of disease.

VITAMIN SAFETY

Vitamins are safer than foods. People die every year from allergic reactions to peanuts and shellfish, and from food poisoning – but no one has ever died from overdosing on vitamins.

Upon rare occasion the press reports on alleged vitamin toxicity, but conspicuously absent are hard scientific data and the names of supposed victims. We never read, for example, "This morning John Doe of Seattle died of an overdose of vitamin C." Why not? Because it has never happened. If it had, it would have made front page news.

Articles condemning the use of vitamins as unsafe are based on fear, not fact. They are merely reports from so-called experts who *believe* that vitamins are harmful, based on personal opinion or on literature they have read. Curiously, many of these vitamin detractors also promote the use of prescription drugs, which are infinitely more harmful (and profitable) than vitamins. What is it that vitamin antagonists really fear – loss of life or loss of income?

According to the 32nd annual report (2016) from the American Association of Poison Control Centers (AAPCC), there were no deaths whatsoever from vitamins in the year 2014 – zero deaths from multiple vitamins, vitamin A, niacin, vitamin B-6, other B-vitamins, vitamin C, vitamin D, vitamin E, or from any vitamin at all. Year after year, decade after decade, the AAPCC reports are boringly always the same: zero deaths from vitamins.

The levels of vitamins normally ingested by the average North American in diet and multi-vitamin supplements are insufficient to produce side effects. The exceedingly rare cases of vitamin toxicity that do occur are reversible and leave no lasting effects. When the vitamin in question is withdrawn, symptoms disappear and the body returns to its previous state.

According to exhaustive review of scientific data, vitamin C is non-toxic, even when taken in very large amounts. Daily oral intakes of up to 6,000 mg. for 15 months and up to 8,000 mg. for 10 days have been administered without any side effects or over-sensitivity reactions. Very large quantities of vitamin C can produce temporary diarrhea and/or excess intestinal gas but, contrary to popular myth – *no* kidney stones, *no* rebound scurvy, *no* gout, and *no* destruction of vitamin B-12 have ever been documented to have been caused by vitamin C excess.

The toxicity of vitamin A has been highly exaggerated. There are five or fewer cases of hypervitaminosis A reported annually and zero deaths from it. Complete withdrawal of vitamin A results in disappearance of symptoms in a matter of a few days to a few weeks. According to the *Merck Manual* (16th ed.), acute vitamin A toxicity has been observed in children who took over 300,000 IU or adults who took several million IU at one time. Chronic vitamin A toxicity in older children and adults may develop after daily doses above 100,000 IU have been taken for months. Infants may develop signs of toxicity within a few weeks when given from 20,000 to 60,000 IU of *synthetic*, water dispersible vitamin A (which is not as well tolerated as natural, fat-soluble vitamin A). Two cases of adult hepatic injury have been reported, one in a woman who took from 100,000 to 1,250,000 IU daily for five years, the other in a man who took 400,000 IU daily for eight years. All of these amounts are incredibly high, far beyond those provided by any sensible supplement program.

Those whose liver functions has been compromised by drugs, viral hepatitis, alcohol abuse, or protein-calorie malnutrition may have a lower tolerance for vitamin A than those with healthy livers. Many adults have taken over 400,000 IU for several months (e.g., for treatment of acne) without any side effect whatever. One study claims that one million IU taken daily for five years didn't lead to toxicity in a series of patients.

Vitamin D is potentially the most toxic of the vitamins. Massive doses may lead to calcification of soft tissues. According to the *Merck Manual* (16th ed.), 40,000 IU of vitamin D daily may produce toxicity within one to four months in infants. Toxic effects have been observed in adults receiving 100,000 IU daily for several months. (Again, these amounts are astronomical compared to those provided by a sensible program of supplementation.)

Anything can become toxic if we get too much of it – including water, sunshine, and oxygen. Fatal uremia, for example, can be induced by drinking over 12 litres of water daily. Vitamins, however, have an incredibly wide margin of safety. For some, it takes hundreds or thousands of times our normal intake to produce toxicity. For others, no toxic reactions have been found at any level of intake. Consequences of vitamin overdose are temporary and reversible.

Inadequate vitamin intake is more of a threat to public health than the exceedingly rare instances of vitamin toxicity. Brush aside the smoke screen of anecdote, hearsay, exaggeration, and fear in order to help yourself to better health.

VITAMIN A DEFICIENCY

The myths about vitamin A toxicity have scared many people into taking much less than their bodies need, or none at all. The human liver is capable of storing up to 500,000 I.U. of vitamin A. Yet on autopsy, many adult livers are found to contain zero vitamin A. Symptoms of vitamin A deficiency are rampant in our culture and include: poor night vision, eyes sensitive to glare, conjunctivitis, sinus problems, acne, and warts. From 20,000 to 40,000 I.U. of supplemental vitamin A (palmitate) is probably what many adults require for optimal health.

ZINC DEFICIENCY

Insufficient zinc can cause loss of taste or smell, anorexia, prostate problems, or low sperm counts. Zinc deficiency sometimes shows up as white spots under the fingernails. Daily supplementation with 30 mg. of zinc (gluconate or citrate) is a wise preventative measure. Therapeutically, zinc needs to be taken in the range of from 50 to 75 mg. daily.

VITAMIN B-6 DEFICIENCY

Carpal tunnel syndrome is characterized by the inability to close one's hand into a tight fist. There may be numbness, pain, prickling, or tingling affecting some part of the median nerve distribution of the hand (palmar side of the thumb, index finger, radial half of ring finger, radial half of the palm). In the absence of traumatic injury to the wrist, all of the above are symptoms of a vitamin B-6 deficiency.

Nausea and vomiting of pregnancy is caused by a vitamin B-6 deficiency. So is abruptio placenta, the spontaneous premature detachment of a normally situated placenta after the 20th week of gestation.

All of the above conditions can be prevented by taking at least 50 mg. of vitamin B-6 daily (30 times the RDA), in conjunction with similar amounts of the other major B-vitamins. Therapeutically, it may take 100 mg. per day of B-6 to correct carpal tunnel syndrome.

IODINE DEFICIENCY

Breast lumps may be caused by iodine deficiency. A number of studies show that women with low iodine intake have symptoms relating to severe hyperplasia and fibrocystic disease of the breast that can subsequently be corrected by iodine replacement. No one really knows how much iodine the body needs for optimal functioning. The RDA of 15 mcg. per day is probably based on slightly more than the amount required to eliminate goitre and cretinism in the general population. Doses averaging 5,000 mcg. of iodine per day (300 times the RDA) have been shown to dissolve benign cystic breast lumps, and that amount may also be a good preventative level to take. Vitamin E (600 I.U. daily) assists iodine in the protection of breast tissue.

CALCIUM AND MAGNESIUM

Spurs or pointed projections sticking out from bones are caused by too much calcium – correct? Wrong. The opposite is true. Bone spurs are caused by deficiencies of both calcium and magnesium. The blood requires calcium so desperately that in emergencies it robs the bones to get it. If this calcium is not soluble, some of it precipitates out at the bone sites from which it is taken. What keeps calcium in solution is magnesium.

Spontaneous muscle cramps in the calf, foot, upper thighs, low back, or hands are caused by deficiencies or imbalances in calcium and magnesium. Arrhythmia (irregular heartbeat) is often caused by deficiencies or imbalances in calcium and magnesium.

Startle reactions, hypersensitivity to noise (hyperreflexia), restless legs, and repeated tapping of hands and feet are symptoms of a magnesium deficiency. Cravings for chocolate (except for allergic addiction) can also be symptomatic of a magnesium deficiency.

All of the above problems tend to be aggravated by diets high in sugar and caffeine, both of which factors deplete calcium. Daily supplementation with calcium (800 mg.), magnesium (500 mg.), potassium (400 mg.), and vitamin D (200 I.U.) usually bring complete relief from all of the above. Potassium is an electrolyte co-partner to calcium and magnesium. Vitamin D helps the body to make efficient use of calcium.

MYTHS ABOUT VITAMIN TOXICITY

Vitamin A and birth defects: A number of birth defects have been reported in children born to mothers who had been taking isotretinoin for their acne. Isotretinoin (*aka* etretinate, accutane) is a synthetic derivative of an artificial (adulterated) form of vitamin A, that was available by prescription only. No birth defects have been reported in mothers who took dietary supplements of natural vitamin A from fish liver oils. [Question: *Why would anyone promote a synthetic drug for acne relief when natural vitamin A is just as effective and a whole lot safer?* Answer: *You can't make much money from selling an unpatentable vitamin.*]

Vitamin C and Kidney Stones: There is no scientific data to support the belief that vitamin C might cause kidney stones. Many studies have found that large daily intakes of vitamin C (e.g., in excess of 6,000 mg.) neither increase urinary oxalate excretion nor increase the incidence of kidney stones. The supposed "evidence" linking vitamin C in this matter is anecdotal. A letter to the editor of the *Lancet* (July 28, 1973) claims to have found a high oxalate output in one person who ingested vitamin C for seven days. No kidney stones were produced, only the speculative fear that they might be. A second letter to the editor (Dec. 22, 1973) was written by a doctor who had heard from an associate (i.e., by *hearsay*) that someone had passed a urinary stone after taking 2,000 mg. of vitamin C for only two weeks. [Note: *Not everything that appears in medical journals is necessarily scientific. Unsubstantiated letters to the editor are in the category of "anecdotal evidence" rather than documented fact.*]

Rebound Scurvy: It has been rumoured for decades that adults who take large amounts of vitamin C may develop scurvy if they reduce those levels drastically, or that infants born to mothers taking large amounts of vitamin C may be born with scurvy. There is no scientific data to support this notion. There were two speculative reports to this effect, but the diagnoses were not confirmed by clinical chemistry: no plasma vitamin C levels were reported, and the time for the onset of alleged symptoms was suspiciously short. On the other hand, two studies showed that excessive intake of vitamin C does *not* result in blood levels lower than normal.

Vitamin B-6 and Nerve Damage: In 1983, the *New England Journal of Medicine* (309:445) published a report about six patients who took from 2,000 to 6,000 mg. of vitamin B-6 daily for up to 40 months and who developed peripheral sensory neuropathy. Symptoms included muscular incoordination, unsteady gait, difficulty handling small objects, sensory changes in lips and tongue, diminished reflexes, and reduced sensations of touch in the upper and lower limbs. (According to the *Merck Manual*, such sensory neuropathy is reversible on cessation of the B-6.) This was not a controlled study but an account of six case histories. We do not know, for example, how many people took similar amounts of B-6 without experiencing any adverse effects at all. Also, these same symptoms can also be caused by deficiencies of vitamin B-1 and/or magnesium. This controversial report drew considerable flak from readers. The author of the study responded with a letter to the editor stating that he had also found one patient who took only 500 mg. of vitamin B-6 daily for one year and developed "the sensation of electric shocks shooting down her spine after neck flexion." Such a symptom, however, is characteristic of a vitamin B-12 deficiency (or even a chiropractic misalignment of neck vertebrae).

Vitamin B-6 needs to be taken in balance with its co-partners (e.g., magnesium, and other B-vitamins). To take one of these by itself can produce deficiencies in others. This is simply imbalance, not toxicity. [Question: *Seven reports are not enough to determine the efficacy of any vitamin. How can they be enough to establish any alleged toxicity?*]

NATURAL AND SYNTHETIC

Natural ingredients in food supplements are preferable to synthetic ones, are they not? The most accurate answer is "sometimes". We need to define our terms very carefully.

Natural means "existing in or produced by nature." Synthetic means "manufactured." In a certain sense, no tablets or capsules are natural. They do not grow on trees. All supplements are manufactured; the question is from which materials.

To further complicate matters, the human body does a lot of synthesizing of its own. It synthesizes proteins from amino acids, niacin from tryptophan, and vitamin D from the action of sunlight on cholesterol under the skin. All animals and plants take certain raw materials and convert or naturally synthesize them into other essential substances. Synthesis in a laboratory can sometimes also be an entirely natural process.

Humans cannot manufacture vitamin C (ascorbate) in their livers the way that animals do. The vitamin C that is produced commercially, however, is made from glucose outside the body in exactly the same way that animals make it from glucose in their livers, by subjecting it to the very same enzyme: L-gulonolactone oxidase. Is the end result natural or synthetic? Clearly, it is both. The resulting ascorbate molecule manufactured commercially is identical to the one animals produce naturally within their bodies.

The problem in comparing "natural" to "synthetic" is that the two terms are not opposites. They can overlap. The correct opposite of "natural" is "artificial." Everything we eat or drink, including water, is a chemical. Natural chemicals are those that our bodies need. Artificial chemicals are those that are foreign to the body. Synthetic chemicals are those produced in a laboratory, and they can be either natural or artificial.

Natural sources of water-soluble vitamins are both unreliable and of low yield for manufacturing supplements. Brewer's yeast is the richest natural source of B-vitamins, yet a whole tablespoonful contains on average only about 1.25 mg. of thiamine (B-1), 0.34 mg. of riboflavin (B-2), and 3 mg. of niacin. This content can fluctuate widely from batch to batch, making it difficult to maintain consistent label claims. Also, many people have sensitivities to yeasts and would do better not to consume products from this source.

In order to comply with the strict rules regarding the potency of vitamin products, manufactures use crystalline vitamins. A crystalline vitamin is a natural one that may have originally been isolated from a food source but now appears in its purest, most refined form – without any traces of the original food remaining. Even low potency formulations use crystalline vitamins in order to meet standards of uniformity.

All manufacturers of vitamin and formulations – including those who claim *not* to use "synthetic" vitamins – buy their raw materials from the same suppliers. There are very few original sources of ingredients. In all of North America, for example, there is only one reliable manufacturer of the vitamin C that is used in making supplements.

Labels can be deceiving. "Rose hips" vitamin C tablets, for example, often reveal a content of only five percent rose hips powder. The balance is pure ascorbic acid. Rose hips contain only a tiny percentage of ascorbate, and from 45 to 90 percent of that may be lost during the drying process. To provide 1,000 mg. of vitamin C entirely from rose hips, the tablet would have to be the size of a baseball and would cost hundreds of dollars per bottle. Herbal sources are both too expensive and too unreliable for the potency that the body needs.

Acerola cherries are the richest known source of vitamin C existing in nature. Yet, they contain only about 1.6 percent of vitamin C by weight. Those manufacturers who claim to use vitamin C only from acerola are not telling the truth. They use the same manufactured source of vitamin C that everyone else does, with only a dash of acerola powder added.

As long as we are talking about water-soluble vitamins (C and the B-complex), it does not matter where the vitamin comes from – whether directly from a plant or from a laboratory. The resultant molecule is identical and is handled by the body in exactly the same way. In other words, vitamin C extracted from rose hips and vitamin C synthesized from corn starch are identical in their pure form.

Where vitamin C occurs in plants (such as rose hips and acerola cherries) it does so together with a group of related compounds known as bioflavonoids. These substances have effects on the body similar to those from vitamin C and they may provide some synergy with respect to the body's utilization of vitamin C. That is the reason that many manufacturers add bioflavonoids to their vitamin C products. This additional feature does not change the fact that the vitamin C content itself is both synthetic and natural. It is interesting to note that animals make vitamin C in their livers but they do not make bioflavonoids. It appears that bioflavonoids may be useful but not essential to mammals.

There are differences, however, in the structures of the natural and synthetic versions of the fat soluble vitamins, A, D and E. The various forms are physically different when viewed under a microscope and they are handled differently by the body. In this case, the synthetic versions are artificial.

Evidence strongly suggests that vitamins A and D are more toxic in their synthetic (artificial) form than in their natural versions. There is no evidence of toxicity from synthetic (artificial) vitamin E; however, it does not seem to be utilized as efficiently as its natural counterpart.

Natural is definitely the best way to go for nutritional supplements, but sometimes natural and synthetic are one and the same. It is artificial vitamins (not necessarily synthetic) that the body does not handle well.

CHELATED MINERALS

Chelation is the natural process by which the body absorbs inorganic minerals. During the digestion of a meal, proteins are broken down into their constituent amino acids; and inorganic mineral compounds are separated into positively and negatively charged ions. Some of the free amino acids surround (chelate) the mineral ions, thereby neutralizing their electrical charges. Without an electrical charge, the chelated minerals slip easily through the negatively charged intestinal wall without either sticking to it or being repelled by it.

For chelation to work well, two conditions have to be met: (1) proteins and minerals need to be in the stomach at the same time. (2) the stomach has to have adequate levels of hydrochloric acid. Thus, it is best to take mineral supplements with meals, when the stomach is actively producing acid and when protein molecules are also present.

Some manufacturers produce supplements in which the minerals are pre-chelated with amino acids. These chelated minerals are readily absorbed between meals and by those with digestive weaknesses. By taking supplements with meals, however, a person with adequate digestion receives no benefit from taking pre-chelated minerals.

A person with weak digestion who takes chelated minerals is bypassing a serious underlying problem. If someone cannot absorb non-chelated minerals from supplements, that person will also have difficulty absorbing them from food. It makes more sense to support the digestive weakness by taking supplementary hydrochloric acid and digestive enzymes with meals. In that way the body will be better able to absorb minerals (and all other factors) from meals as well as from supplements.

Chelated mineral supplements are both expensive and unnecessary. They have another disadvantage: they are low potency. Amino acid chelates characteristically contain only from one to 10 percent of the elemental mineral in question. Conventional (i.e., non-chelated) mineral compounds have a much higher content. Calcium carbonate, for example, is 40 percent calcium; magnesium oxide is 60 percent magnesium.

Proponents often claim that, because of better absorption, the lower potency chelates are more effective than higher potency conventional minerals. This might be the case only if taken between meals by someone with weak digestion – in which case it makes more sense to support the digestive weakness rather than to bypass it.

WHAT ELSE IS INCLUDED

Labels are usually detailed about the active ingredients in a formula and vague about its non-active fillers, sweeteners, and excipients. (An excipient is any substance added to a powder so that it can be formed into a tablet of the proper shape and consistency.)

Chewable tablets have a high sugar content. It is not possible to make a multi-vitamin tablet palatable without adding an incredible amount of sweetener of some kind. Minerals and B-vitamins, especially, taste terrible in their pure forms. Some manufacturers dance around the issue by declaring that their chewables contain fructose, concentrated fruit juice, honey, or the like; but all of these are concentrated sugars. They have the same effects on dental caries, hypoglycemia, and diabetes as any other form of sugar.

CAPSULES AND TABLETS

Many supplements are available in gelatin capsules, some of which are from vegetable sources. Capsules have four limitations. (1) They tend to spill their contents into the digestive tract all at one place. This could be a problem if some of the contents are potentially irritating to the mucosa of the stomach or intestines. (2) They do not prevent interactions between ingredients. Therefore, they can be used only for simple formulas where there are no ingredients that can react with each other. (3) Ingredients in capsules cannot be compressed; therefore, it takes more capsules than tablets to deliver the same quantity of nutrients. (4) Capsules tend to cost more than tablets.

Tablets break down more gradually in the intestinal tract, they are less expensive to make, they make it possible to separate ingredients that might otherwise interact, and their ingredients are compressed. The disadvantage of tablets is that more excipients have to be added during the manufacturing process than for capsules.

A SENSIBLE PROGRAM

For most adults without significant health problems, a sensible supplement program needs to include a high potency, balanced, broad-spectrum formula that provides 12 vitamins and 12 minerals – plus an extra 1,000 mg. of vitamin C daily. Such a buffet of nutrients offers potential support for every link in the vitamin-mineral chain.

Protein supplements are not usually necessary for optimal health. Except for extreme dietary fads, insufficient protein intake is rarely a problem in the western world. Digestive weakness is very common, however. Many people are unable to break down and utilize the proteins that they eat. Almost everyone over 40 would benefit from taking a broad spectrum digestive enzyme supplement with meals – especially one that includes betaine hydrochloride, pepsin, pancreatin, bile, and papain.

Most westerners consume far more fat in total than they need, and usually of the wrong kind. Some health conscious people attempt to reduce dietary fats down to dangerously low levels, in a mistaken belief that all fats are bad. There is a balance, and that balance may include supplements of essential fatty acids (e.g., fish body oil concentrates, organic flaxseed oil).

Food supplementation is an individual matter. What is optimal for one person may be too little for some and too much for others. People with specific health concerns may need to pay extra attention to certain factors.

CHOOSING A MULTI-VITAMIN

The information below comes from decades of experience in formulating high potency natural source dietary supplements. Textbook explanations vary from incomplete fragments to overwhelming details, many of which are irrelevant to health consumers. Promotional literature tends to focus on partial truths that make one supplier's product appear to be superior to others. However complex nutritional biochemistry may be, it can be reduced to simple basic principles. Once you understand which molecules are natural to the human body, everything else falls into place. With the guidelines below, you will be able to read the label of any vitamin-mineral product and have an instant sense of whether or not it is really what you wish for yourself.

OPTIMAL AMOUNTS

One-per-day multi-vitamins typically provide little more than enough key ingredients to prevent advanced deficiency diseases (e.g., scurvy, beri beri, pellagra, goitre, rickets) – a poor insurance plan at best. Optimal health requires taking specific nutrients in much higher potencies than the tiny amounts suggested by published tables. Adults who are not satisfied with minimal nutrition are well advised to take the following amounts of supplementary vitamins, minerals and lipotropic factors daily, within the ranges suggested below. [Note: *these are not necessarily therapeutic levels. Those with atherosclerosis, diabetes, and other degenerative conditions may need much higher amounts of some factors.*]

Nutrient	Low Optimum	High Optimum*
Vitamin A (palmitate)	10,000 I.U.	12,000 I.U.
Vitamin D-3	800 I.U.	800 I.U.
Vitamin E (D-alpha)	400 I.U.	600 I.U.
Vitamin C (ascorbic acid)	1,500 mg.	2,200 mg.
Vitamin B-1 (thiamine)	50 mg.	100 mg.
Vitamin B-2 (riboflavin)	50 mg.	100 mg.
Niacinamide (B-3)	50 mg.	100 mg.
Pantothenic Acid (B-5)	100 mg.	1,300 mg.
Vitamin B-6	50 mg.	100 mg.
Folic Acid (B-9)	1,000 mcg.	1,200 mcg.
Vitamin B-12	300 mcg.	600 mcg.
Biotin	100 mcg.	220 mcg.
Choline	100 mg.	220 mg.
Inositol	50 mg.	100 mg.
Calcium	800 mg.	800 mg.
Magnesium	500 mg.	500 mg.
Potassium	400 mg.	400 mg.
Iron	20 mg.	22 mg.
Manganese	15 mg.	22 mg.
Zinc	25 mg.	33 mg.
Silicon	20 mg.	22 mg.
Iodine	800 mcg.	2,100 mcg.
Chromium	200 mcg.	330 mcg.
Selenium	200 mcg.	220 mcg.
Molybdenum	20 mcg.	22 mcg.
Vanadium	10 mcg.	12 mcg.

High optimal range is recommended for those with stressful lifestyles or who are hypoglycemic or have allergic tendencies.

It is not possible to fit all of the above ingredients into a single tablet that can be swallowed. Therefore, look for a product that divides the above quantities into from 5 to 8 homogeneous tablets.

OPTIMAL ABSORPTION

The most efficient way to take multi-vitamins is in divided amounts with meals (*e.g., 3 with breakfast, 2 with supper – or 2 with breakfast, 2 with lunch, 1 with supper*). In this way, your body has multiple opportunities to assimilate what it needs, as it is able. Taking all five tablets at once may overwhelm your body with more than it can process, thus wasting a percentage of the nutrients for which you have paid good money.

Optimal absorption requires taking vitamins and minerals with meals. The hydrochloric acid secreted by the stomach in order to digest food also facilitates the breakdown of mineral compounds. In addition, the nutrients in the meal and the nutrients in the tablets act as co-partners, supporting each other.

How the body absorbs minerals (from both food and supplements) is by chelating them internally. Hydrochloric acid in the stomach facilitates the breakdown of mineral compounds into positively and negatively charged ions. The intestinal wall, however, has a mild negative charge: positive ions tend to stick to it rather than be absorbed. To the rescue come amino acids (from protein foods) which surround these mineral ions, neutralizing their electromagnetic charges and facilitating their absorption through the intestinal wall. If you take your mineral supplements with meals, expensive pre-chelated minerals are never needed. Your body does its own chelating.

BIOAVAILABILITY

Bioavailability is a term that comes to us from pharmacology and is often misunderstood when applied to nutrients. The strict definition of bioavailability is "the rate at which a drug is absorbed by the body or exerts its effect after absorption". In practice, this is usually interpreted as the amount of unchanged drug that reaches systemic circulation. When administered intravenously, the bioavailability of any drug is obviously 100 percent.

When applied to dietary supplements, bioavailability usually refers to the percentage of a given vitamin or mineral that can be measured in the blood after ingestion – in other words, how much of a particular dose that is actually absorbed. Such measurements, however, are fraught with limitations.

Absorption of supplementary nutrients is affected by a number of critical factors, including (1) digestive weakness, (2) whether the nutrient is taken with meals or in between, (3) whether the nutrient is taken by itself or as part of a formula that also includes co-partners, and (4) how long after ingestion were the blood measurements taken. Nutrients are most efficiently utilized by the body when accompanied by co-operating synergistic nutrients, when taken with meals when stomach acid is at its peak, and they also tend to trickle into the blood over time. Drugs, on the other hand, tend to bypass normal digestive processes and enter the blood very quickly, regardless of who consumes them. It is unrealistic to apply the absorption standards of drugs to nutrients, which behave in the body in an entirely different way.

Whenever you are presented with a study which suggests that one form of a nutrient has a higher bioavailability, ask who paid for that research. Most of the time it will be a company trying to gain a marketing exclusive for a product that cannot be patented.

Bioavailability research suffers from a number of limitations, the chief one being the digestive ability of the participants in the study. Digestive ability declines with age. The older the participants, the less able they are to absorb anything nutritional. If everyone in the study were given supplementary digestive enzymes, the results of bioavailability studies would be very different.

Bioavailability studies can also be misleading in that the participants may not be typical of the general population (selection bias) – or there aren't enough of them in the study to be able to reach meaningful conclusions (statistical insignificance) – or no measure has been made of how many of the results could have happened by chance (inadequate coefficient of correlation).

Studies such as the above are misused, for example, to claim that magnesium glycinate is more bioavailable than magnesium oxide. Balderdash. Magnesium glycinate provides only 18 percent magnesium, compared to magnesium oxide's 60 percent magnesium. When either compound reaches a stomach that is in the process of digesting food, exactly the same thing happens: (a) hydrochloric acid separates the mineral compound into positive and negatively charged ions, (b) amino acids from the digesting meal surround the magnesium ion, thus neutralizing its positive charge, and (c) this neutral charge enables the magnesium to pass readily through the intestinal wall, which has a slight negative charge. This process is called "chelation", and it is how your body absorbs all of the mineral compounds you consume, from whatever source.

NATURAL SOURCES

Every ingredient in your mult-vitamin-mineral should consist of natural molecules that are bio-compatible with your body. It is not easy to tell which ingredients are natural and which are artificial, because most have chemical sounding names. The following examples may be helpful.

VITAMIN A

Retinol is the chemical name for natural vitamin A. Vitamin A palmitate (retinol palmitate) is the natural source raw material use in making vitamin supplements. Artificial vitamin A has a high potential for toxicity; however, the natural form is quite safe. There have been zero documented cases of harm in adults taking up to 100,000 IU of natural vitamin A daily.

BETA CAROTENE

Beta carotene consists of two molecules of vitamin A (retinol) bonded together. Vitamin A cannot be utilized from beta carotene until the liver enzymatically breaks this bond. Most diabetics and some people with hypothyroidism are unable to convert beta carotene into retinol. If you are diabetic or suspect that you have low thyroid function, you are well advised to get your supplementary vitamin A from retinol palmitate rather than beta carotene.

B-VITAMINS

B-vitamins should be natural, pure microcrystalline vitamins ultimately derived from plant or fungal sources and standardized to ensure potency. Examples include thiamine hydrochloride, thiamine mononitrate, riboflavin, niacin, niacinamide, calcium pantothenate, pyridoxine hydrochloride, cobalamin, cyanocobalamin, folic acid, and biotin.

VITAMIN C

Ascorbic acid is made from plant sources and is bio-identical to the ascorbate molecule produced in the livers of mammals and birds. It is made in exactly the same way that animals do, by exposing glucose to the same enzyme, L-gulonolactone oxidase.

It is the ascorbate molecule that the body needs to support its biochemistry. Ascorbic acid (hydrogen ascorbate) is the most commonly available form of vitamin C and is only mildly acidic – negligible acidity when combined with multiple other ingredients in a multi formula. Buffered forms of vitamin C (e.g., calcium ascorbate, magnesium ascorbate) are non-acidic and are more easily tolerated by those with hypersensitive digestive tracts. If ascorbic acid does not produce any form of gastric distress, then buffered forms of vitamin C are not worth the extra expense.

Plant sources of the ascorbate also provide flavonoid co-partners (e.g., bioflavonoids, hesperidin, rutin, proanthocyanidins). These flavonoids support the action of ascorbate – the reason why some multi formulas also include citrus bioflavonoids. However, animals that produce ascorbate in their livers produce only vitamin C and no flavonoids. It is the ascorbate molecule that the human body requires in large amounts to compensate for its hypoascorbemia.

Acerola cherries are the richest plant source of vitamin C – yet provide only 1.6 percent ascorbate by dry weight. Some companies may claim that their vitamin C is entirely from acerola. This is pure fiction. A tablet containing only 100 mg. of vitamin C from acerola would weigh over 13 pounds (6 kilograms).

Other fiction is the claim that the body utilizes vitamin C from plant sources more efficiently than it does from vitamin C made in a laboratory. Not so. All the body requires is the ascorbate molecule, regardless of its source. The ascorbate produced in a laboratory (from glucose) is bioidentical to the ascorbate produced from glucose in the livers of mammals that do so.

VITAMIN D

Vitamin D-3 (cholecalciferol) is the natural form of vitamin D, bioidentical to the same molecule produced by the action of sunlight on cholesterol under the skin. Natural vitamin D is safe in any amount that can be put into a tablet or capsule. The artificial form of this vitamin (D-2) has a greater potential for toxicity, especially when taken in water-dispersible forms that bypass the liver's ability to monitor its uptake.

VITAMIN E

There are two natural forms of vitamin E: D-alpha tocopherol (fat soluble) and D-alpha tocopheryl succinate (water dispersible). The artificial forms of vitamin E (DL-alpha), while harmless, are less efficiently utilized by the body.

CHELATED MINERALS

Chelated minerals (e.g., proteinates, HVP chelates) are best used in multi formulas for micro-minerals (e.g., chromium, selenium, vanadium) because this is the most efficient delivery system for minerals required in tiny amounts. Chelated minerals typically provide only about 5 percent of the mineral in question; the other 95 percent being taken up by the amino acids that do the chelating. Using a powder that has 20 times the volume of the isolated micro-mineral ensures that it will be blended uniformly with other ingredients that are present in much larger amounts.

ORGANIC MINERALS

Organic mineral compounds are those which contain carbon in their molecular structure (e.g., gluconates, fumarates, picolinates, orotates). Organic mineral molecules are bonded together by co-valence and have a neutral electromagnetic charge that enables them to pass readily through the intestinal wall (which has a slight negative charge). Inorganic forms of iron (e.g., chloride, sulphate) tend to stick to the intestinal wall, causing poor absorption and constipation. Organic iron compounds (e.g., fumarate, gluconate) do not do this.

INORGANIC MINERALS

Some minerals are efficiently utilized by the body in their inorganic form ("inorganic" meaning that they do not have carbon in their molecular structure). These include the electrolyte minerals (calcium, magnesium, potassium) as well as iodine, silicon, and chloride. Inorganic minerals are bonded by ionic valence and separate into positive and negative ions when broken down by hydrochloric acid in the stomach. Amino acids surround (chelate) the ions, facilitating their absorption through the intestinal wall. The body uses positively charged calcium, magnesium, and potassium ions – plus negatively charged chloride ions – as electrolytes to regulate fluid pressures, the flow of nerve impulses, and pH balance throughout the body.

CALCIUM CARBONATE

Calcium carbonate is one of three natural forms of calcium found in human bones (the others being calcium phosphate and hydroxyapatite). Calcium carbonate is also the natural form found in oyster shell and coral calcium, two highly promoted supplements. Calcium carbonate provides approximately 40 percent calcium, making it the most efficient natural source to use in supplements. (Calcium lactate, for example, provides only 15 percent calcium and chelated forms of calcium about 5 percent.) If you take your calcium carbonate supplements with meals, they are just as well absorbed as any other form of calcium.

MAGNESIUM OXIDE

The magnesium oxide molecule provides approximately 60 percent magnesium, making it the most efficient natural source of magnesium to use in supplements. If you take your magnesium oxide supplements with meals, they are just as well absorbed as any other form of magnesium.

CHLORIDE MOLECULES

The body utilizes chloride molecules from vitamin and mineral compounds (a) to manufacture stomach acid (hydrochloric acid), and (b) as an electrolyte to help regulate fluid pressures and the flow of nerve impulses. Thus, it is helpful if some of the ingredients in your multi formula provide the chloride molecule (e.g., betaine hydrochloride, potassium chloride, thiamine hydrochloride, pyridoxine hydrochloride).

TIMED RELEASE VITAMINS

The timed release of vitamins is one of those ideas that works better in theory than in practise. During the manufacturing process, blended powders are segregated into several groups. Layers of a waxy coating are applied in varying thicknesses: one group receives no coating, a second group receives one layer, a third group receives two layers, and so on. The assumption is that digestive juices take time to work through the various layers of wax, progressively releasing vitamins as they go. Problem: there are only so many feet of digestive tract through which vitamins can be absorbed and only so much time in which it can be done. Those vitamins that are released in the right place at the right time can be absorbed; but if a person's digestion is weak, most of the vitamins will end up in the toilet bowel. It makes more sense to take normal vitamins two or three times per day than it does to invest in the timed release concept.

EXCIPIENTS

Every vitamin-mineral tablet has to contain a small percentage of excipients. These are inert extra ingredients needed to help powders flow freely through the machinery, to prevent raw tablets from sticking to the compression dies, and to ensure the integrity of the final tablet. Examples of completely natural excipients are cellulose, magnesium stearate (from plant sources), stearic acid (from animal sources), di-calcium phosphate, croscarmellose sodium, hydroxypropyl cellulose, hypromellose, and silicon dioxide.

HYPO-ALLERGENIC

Low potency supplements may contain fillers such as lactose, corn starch, potato starch, flour, soy derivatives, or various kinds of sugars. These substances can trigger allergic reactions in those who are sensitive to them. Fillers are needed when the active ingredients are not of sufficient volume to fill the capsules or tableting dies. With high potency vitamin-mineral products there is rarely a need for fillers. When there is, responsible manufacturers use innocuous di-calcium phosphate rather than the potentially allergenic options.

ANEMIA

Anemia is any condition in which the hemoglobin content of the blood is less than required to meet the oxygen demands of the body. Symptoms can include pale skin, fingernail beds, and mucous membranes; sore tongue; drowsiness; general malaise; difficult breathing; gastrointestinal disturbances; loss of libido; and diminished menstrual flow.

Iron deficiency anemia results from a greater demand on stored iron than can be supplied. The red blood cell count may be normal, but there will be insufficient hemoglobin. Erythrocytes will be pale and have abnormal shapes. This is probably the most common chronic disease of human kind. It is caused by inadequate iron intake, malabsorption of iron, chronic blood loss, pregnancy and lactation, the destruction of hemoglobin cellular membranes, or a combination of these factors.

Heme is the iron-containing non-protein portion of the hemoglobin molecule, wherein iron is in its ferrous (water soluble) state. Iron found in plant sources is predominantly in its ferric (insoluble) state. This means that the heme iron from animal sources is readily absorbed and utilized by the body, whereas plant sources of iron are not. For this reason, vegetarian diets increase the risk of iron deficiency anemia.

A number of nutritional deficiencies are usually involved, including vitamin C, iron, and the B-complex vitamins, especially B-12 & Folic Acid. A hydrochloric acid deficiency also prevents iron from being absorbed from the diet. Ferrous forms of iron supplements (e.g., fumarate, gluconate) are readily absorbed. Ferric iron (e.g., chloride, sulphate) is poorly absorbed and causes constipation.

Pernicious anemia is an advanced form of vitamin B-12 deficiency characterized by weakness, sore tongue, tingling and numbness of the extremities, and gastrointestinal symptoms (e.g., diarrhea, nausea, vomiting, pain). Pernicious anemia occurs when the parietal cells of the stomach lining fail to secrete enough intrinsic factor to ensure intestinal absorption of vitamin B-12 (the extrinsic factor). This is due to atrophy of the glandular mucosa of the fundus of the stomach and is associated with absence of hydrochloric acid (achlorhydria).

Nutritional treatment involves (a) taking high dose natural vitamin B-12 (either cyanocobalamin or cobalamin) under the tongue (sublingually), and (b) taking digestive enzyme supplements that provide generous amounts of hydrochloric acid (in a stable form, such as betaine hydrochloride). In cases where the nutritional protocol may not be enough, intramuscular injections of vitamin B-12 are required.

Folic acid anemia is, as its name suggests, anemia resulting from a deficiency of folic acid – a vitamin factor found primarily in green leafy vegetables (hence the name "folic" meaning "from foliage") as well as broccoli, asparagus, legumes, nuts, grains, organ meats, and a few fruits.

SUPPLEMENTS FOR ANEMIA

Vitamin B-12 and folic acid are nutritional co-partners. They work together in a number of biochemical processes and have similar symptoms of deficiency. The therapeutic implication of this relationship is that large amounts of supplementary vitamin B-12 can mask a folic acid deficiency, which if untreated, could have serious consequences. For this reason, supplementary B-12 and folic acid should always be taken together, in equal amounts.

Daily supplements that are of benefit to the above anemias are sublingual **vitamin B-12** (2,000 mcg.) with **folic acid** (2,000 mcg.), plus the other major **B-vitamins** (50 mg. of each), **vitamin C** (2,000 mg.), **ferrous fumarate** (20 mg.), and digestive enzyme formulas providing **betaine hydrochloride.**

OSTEOPOROSIS

Osteoporosis is a reduction in the mass of bones. About 98.5 percent of the calcium in the human body is found in the bones and teeth. Most of the remaining 1.5 percent is required by the bloodstream, on a high priority basis. If the blood does not get enough calcium, it takes what it needs from the bones. Blood tests often show normal levels of calcium during osteoporosis.

Bone spurs and calcification of tissues are caused by deficiencies of both calcium and magnesium. When the bloodstream takes calcium from the bones, if there is also not enough magnesium to keep this calcium soluble, some of it precipitates out to leave spurs at the sites from which it was taken.

It is not necessary to consume dairy products in order to get enough calcium. Calcium is widely dispersed throughout our food supply. It is found in tiny amounts in almost every food and in significant amounts in almonds, barley, beet greens, dates, filberts, kale, molasses, mustard greens, oysters, peanuts, salmon, sardines, soy, spinach, sunflower seeds, turnip greens, and English walnuts. Cows don't drink milk, yet they have plenty of dietary calcium to put into their milk. They get it from the greens they eat. So can we. There are many Asian, African and other cultures which do not consume dairy products at all yet have an extremely low incidence of osteoporosis.

Lack of calcium in the bones may have less to do with low intake than it has to do with calcium-depleting factors in our lifestyle. Sugar causes the body to deplete calcium. Caffeine (coffee, tea, colas) also causes the body to deplete calcium. When both sugar and caffeine are consumed together, they have a multiplier effect on the amount of calcium depleted. Excessive phosphorus (e.g., in soft drinks) also causes the body to waste calcium. So does lack of exercise.

Calcium in the bones occurs as three different compounds: calcium phosphate, calcium carbonate, and hydroxyapatite. Of these, calcium carbonate is the most efficient source to use in dietary supplements.

Even if dietary intake of calcium is sufficient, the body has to have enough of certain other factors in order to be able to utilize that calcium. Magnesium is needed to keep calcium in solution, to keep it from precipitating out to form bone spurs and kidney stones. High potassium intake is associated with low calcium excretion. Vitamin D is needed by the parathyroid glands to regulate calcium metabolism. Silicon acts as a catalyst for calcium utilization.

In addition to their roles in bone building, calcium, magnesium, and potassium are electrolyte minerals that the body requires in balance – to help regulate fluid pressures, transmit nerve impulses, and contract muscles. Supplementation with calcium-magnesium-potassium in the ratio of 8:5:4 also helps to relieve hypertension, insomnia, irregular heartbeat, irritability, muscle cramps/spasms, nervous tics/twitches, and hypersensitivity to noise.

STRENGTHEN DIGESTION

Weak digestion contributes significantly to osteoporosis. There has to be enough hydrochloric acid in the stomach to break down calcium compounds. There has to be enough bile to emulsify fats into droplets tiny enough to be acted upon by lipase (fat-splitting) enzymes. Gall bladder insufficiency causes large globules of fat to remain in the gut, attracting calcium and other minerals (electromagnetically) to form insoluble soaps that cannot be absorbed through the intestinal wall – and is thus a major contributor to mineral deficiencies of every kind. Everyone with osteoporosis needs to take broad spectrum digestive enzyme support that includes both betaine hydrochloride and bile salts.

OSTEO SUPPORT

Osteoporosis can be overcome by paying attention to all of the factors involved: (1) restrict sugar, caffeine, and soft drinks, (2) exercise regularly, (3) support digestive function with a broad spectrum enzyme formula that includes **betaine hydrochloride** and **bile**, (4) ensure that total daily intake of **vitamin D** is at least 2,000 I.U., and (5) take the following mineral supplements daily: 800 mg. of **calcium** (from carbonate), 500 mg. of **magnesium** (from oxide), 400 mg. of **potassium** (from chloride), and 20 mg. of **silicon.**

HYPOGLYCEMIA

Low blood sugar (hypoglycemia) can be the "you won't like me when I'm hungry" syndrome. It is a common dysfunction that involves the pancreas, the adrenal glands, and the liver.

Consumption of concentrated sugars or sweets causes blood sugar (glucose) to rise rapidly. The pancreas responds by producing insulin in order to bring blood glucose back to normal levels – which return may be rapid or slow, depending on the activity level of the pancreas. When a drop in blood sugar approaches what the body considers to be a low safety level, the adrenal glands send hormones to the liver – and the pancreas also sends glucagon – both of which stimulate the liver to convert some of its glycogen stores into glucose. If, however, the adrenal glands are weak, glycogen stores have been depleted, or the liver is overworked, the needed increase in blood sugar does not happen in time and ill-effects are felt – especially in the brain, a highly glucose dependent organ.

Although the brain accounts for only about two percent of total body weight, it requires over 60 percent of blood glucose while the body is in a resting state. This is why many symptoms of hypoglcyemia are brain related: irritability, headaches, worrying, anger, agitation, frustration, temper tantrums, anxiety, crying spells, nervousness, shakiness, depression, hyperactivity, brain "fog".

Chronic hypoglycemia takes two forms: reactive and passive. In reactive hypoglycemia, the pancreas overreacts to the initial sugar challenge by producing more insulin than necessary, causing blood sugar levels to plummet quickly. In passive hypoglycemia, blood glucose takes several hours to descend into the alarm zone. Reactive hypoglycemia is a direct and immediate response to anything that causes a sudden increase in blood sugar. Passive hypoglycemia is a response to a gradually diminishing level of blood sugar – which depends on how long it has been since the last meal. What both forms of hypoglycemia have in common are exhausted adrenal glands and a sluggish liver.

Reactive hypoglycemia is triggered by what is eaten. Passive hypoglycemia depends mainly on the timing of when one eats. It is possible, of course, for the same person to have both. In such cases, avoiding sweets bypasses the immediate hypoglycemic reaction, but may result in a similar response much later if the next meal is delayed for too long.

It is not only concentrated sugars that cause untoward increases in blood sugar. Caffeine, tobacco, alcohol and many drugs tend to produce the same effect, by overstimulating the adrenals and liver into converting glycogen into excess levels of blood glucose. Allergies are also common provokers of hypoglycemic responses.

With passive hypoglycaemia, it is not only going a long time without eating that can trigger symptoms – so may heavy exercise or unusual stress. Sometimes a hypoglycemic response does not happen unless more than one of these influences occur at the same time. For example, some hypoglycemics are fine when they haven't eaten for hours and fine when they are rushing to meet a stressful deadline, but if both events happen together they can launch an otherwise mild mannered person into frenzied panic or uncontrollable outbursts of temper.

Hypoglycemia also creates a condition of hypoxemia (too little oxygen) in the tissues, making cells vulnerable to invasion by viruses. This relationship was demonstrated during the polio epidemic of 1949 when North Carolinans reduced their intake of sugar by 90 percent and polio also decreased in that state by 90 percent. The nervous tissue of the young is more vulnerable to low blood sugar than that of the adult, which is why polio was epidemic among children.

Hypoglycemia often leads to addiction. Many people have found that when they start to feel nervous or irritated, or their energy starts to lag – a "fix" of sugar, caffeine, alcohol or tobacco helps them to bounce them back quickly. But the "fix" is only temporary because it directly causes glucose levels to drop again, thus perpetuating the pattern. Some become so skilled at sensing when the crash is about to happen that they intuitively time their fixes to stave off symptoms before they become too severe. Unfortunately, this counterproductive pattern only masks the symptoms of the problem, all the while driving its cause deeper – by subjecting the adrenal glands to constant, relentless stress.

High sugar intake increases oxidative cellular damage, stresses the pancreas and adrenal glands, produces free radicals in excess, and depletes our bodies of minerals such as chromium, potassium, magnesium, zinc and the B-vitamins. Sugar also inhibits immune processes and interferes with the transport of vitamin C.

Symptoms of hypoglycemia can include:

- nervousness, shakiness or headaches relieved by eating.
- irritable if late for a meal or miss a meal.
- irritable before breakfast.
- sudden, strong cravings for sweets, coffee, or alcohol.
- get hungry soon after eating.
- cold hands or feet.
- wake up at night feeling hungry.
- wake up in middle of night and can't go back to sleep.
- asthmatic attacks.

The medical test for hypoglycemia is the glucose tolerance test (GTT). The person is given a solution of glucose to drink. Blood glucose is monitored at baseline and at periodic intervals to see how it responds to the glucose challenge. Medical interpretation of the readings, however, is inconsistent. Some doctors erroneously believe that as long as blood sugar readings stay within a prescribed "normal" range, there is no hypoglycemia present – no matter how much glucose may fluctuate within that range – and not even if the test itself produces headaches, irritability, nervousness or worse. A GTT taken over too short a time period may not be reliable. At least five hours is necessary to detect passive hypoglycemia. Also, a GTT performed in the quiet calm of a waiting room may not provoke the same hypoglycemic response that it would if the person were subjected to the stresses of daily living.

Because of the above limitations, and for reasons of convenience, it is usually more reliable to take one's own glucose readings throughout the day – with the aid of a glucometer that can be purchased at any drug store. Start with a reading upon arising in the morning. Take readings throughout the day, before meals, after meals, between meals, before going to bed – and especially at any time that any mental symptoms may be experienced (e.g., brain "fog", agitation, headaches, irritability, etc.). Plot these numbers on paper to see if you can determine a pattern and a baseline reading of what is normal for you. If either eating something sweet or going without eating for a long time causes your blood sugar to drop below your particular baseline, hypoglycemia is definitely at work. Another conclusive event is if mental symptoms occur only when your glucose is within a particular range.

You don't have to take any blood sugar readings to find out if you have hypoglycemia. If you have any of the symptoms listed above, try the hypoglycemic diet to see if they go away. Go off the diet to see if they come back. Repeat the process. If every time you are on the hypoglycemic diet you are symptom free and if every time you are off it the symptoms return, guess what – you have hypoglycemia. This is what doctors call a "therapeutic diagnosis".

PREMENSTRUAL SYNDROME

In women susceptible to premenstrual syndrome (PMS), the menstrual cycle brings on mood changes – such as depression, anxiety, emotional reactivity, sadness, hopelessness, tension, tearfulness, anger, withdrawal, fatigue, difficulty concentrating, insomnia, food cravings, binge eating, feeling overwhelmed or out of control, decreased interest in activities, or increased interpersonal conflicts. These mood changes may also be accompanied by physical changes – such as breast tenderness, bloating, weight gain, or headaches. All of the symptoms of PMS occur during the last week of the menstrual cycle and diminish within a few days of the onset of menses.

All emotional symptoms of PMS are caused by hypoglycemia induced by adrenal exhaustion. Women with weak adrenal glands become hypoglycemic for part of their monthly cycles. The adrenals are important to coping with stress, regulating blood sugar and producing sex hormones. If these glands are undernourished, they may be able to cope with daily life during most of the month but fail to function normally when the stress of peak female hormone production is added on to all of life's other stresses. PMS can be prevented by following a hypoglycemic diet and supporting the adrenal glands throughout the entire month.

INSOMNIA

Insomnia is spontaneously awakening in the night and finding it difficult to return to sleep again. This form of sleeplessness is a symptom of hypoglycemia, low blood sugar. In a 24-hour cycle one's blood sugar tends to be lowest around two or three AM. The brain becomes disturbed by lack of its fuel (glucose) and awakens its owner. Snacking on sweets or consuming alcohol just before bedtime aggravates this problem by exaggerating the natural rise and fall of blood sugar levels. Eating a high protein food before bedtime is often all that is needed to correct insomnia. Protein foods stay in the digestive tract for a long time and release their glucose content into the bloodstream very slowly, thus helping to maintain stable blood sugar levels.

HYPERACTIVITY

Hyperactivity is a syndrome characterized by restlessness, increased muscular activity, impulsive behavior, short attention span, and inability to concentrate. Another name for this syndrome is attention-deficit hyperactivity disorder (ADHD). This condition may begin in early childhood but may not be diagnosed until after the symptoms have been present for many years.

The mental/behavioral abnormalities of ADHD occur when glucose supply to the brain is diminished – strongly suggesting that hyperactivity is a symptom of hypoglycemia. Two factors cause blood glucose levels to plummet – (1) ingestion of concentrated sugars and sweets, and (2) reactions to hidden food allergies. When all sugary and allergenic foods are completely removed from the diet, hyperactive children's behavior returns to normal – but the elimination must be total. Almost any food can trigger hyperactivity in a sensitive child; and the most common offenders are sugar, milk, aspartame, artificial food dyes and additives, and salicylates. If chewable or liquid vitamins are given to hyperactive children, it is crucial that these preparations contain no hidden sugar of any kind, nor any artificial colorings or sweeteners.

ASTHMA

Asthma is constriction of the bronchial airways characterized by difficult breathing and wheezing, or by fits of coughing. In susceptible people, asthmatic attacks are often precipitated by exposure to inhalant allergens (e.g., dust, mold spores, animal dander), foods (e.g., eggs, shellfish, chocolate), or drugs (e.g., ASA/aspirin compounds). One piece of vital information: every asthmatic is also hypoglycemic. It is impossible to get an asthmatic attack unless blood sugar levels are low. Diabetics, for example, never get asthma – with one rare exception: those with dysinsulinism (fluctuating blood sugar levels) can get asthma when their blood sugar is too low but never when it is in the diabetic range.

Increasing blood sugar levels to normal (i.e., by eating or drinking something sweet) stops an asthmatic attack. The drug inhalers used to dilate the bronchial tubes also stimulate the adrenal glands to release glucose from the liver, thus increasing blood sugar levels. If they didn't do that, they would not be able to stop the attack.

The drop in blood sugar that precedes an asthmatic attack can be brought on by exposure to something to which the person is allergic, by consuming a sugary food or beverage, or by stress. The target organs that make one vulnerable to both allergies and low blood sugar are the adrenal glands. Asthma can be overcome by taking the following three actions: (1) identify and eliminate all inhalant and food allergens, (2) strictly follow a hypoglycemic diet, and (3) strengthen the adrenal glands.

HYPOGLYCEMIC DIET

The hypoglycemic diet requires *totally* eliminating all refined and concentrated sugars, all caffeine (coffee, tea, colas), all alcohol and all tobacco. The diet needs to consist of protein foods (e.g., eggs, fish, poultry, tofu) plus complex carbohydrates (e.g., 100 percent whole grains, legumes, starchy vegetables), green vegetables, and low to moderate amounts of natural fats (e.g., butter, olive oil). All of these foods release their glucose into the bloodstream relatively slowly.

It is also necessary to avoid fruit juices and dried fruits, all of which are high in naturally occurring sugars. The occasional piece of whole, raw, unsweetened fruit, however, may be well tolerated by many hypoglycemics – provided it is eaten shortly before a significant meal. Avoid the temptation to use natural fruits as a substitute "fix" that perpetuates the hypoglycemic cycle.

Passive hypoglycemics may also need to have four or five small meals spread throughout the day rather than the three traditional large ones. These people usually feel hunger in their head before they feel it in their bodies. They often wake up in the night (i.e., when blood sugar levels are lowest) and can't get back to sleep. Solution: before going to bed, have a light protein snack.

ADRENAL SUPPORT

Hypoglycemia exhausts the adrenal glands. Nutrients especially important to the health of the adrenals on a daily basis include **vitamin C** (2,000 mg.), **pantothenic acid** (1,000 mg.), **chromium** (300 mcg.), **magnesium** (500 mg.), **zinc** (30 mg.), plus 100 mg. of each of the major **B-vitamins**.

VIRAL INFECTIONS

Viruses are organisms so tiny that they cannot be seen with an ordinary light microscope. They are invaders that depend on nutrients inside the cells of the host for their metabolic and reproductive needs. They burrow into cells and use the DNA/RNA replication machinery of the host cell to reproduce themselves. When viruses enter cells, they may immediately trigger a disease process or they may lay dormant for many years.

Viruses damage the host cell by blocking its normal protein synthesis and by using its metabolic machinery for their own reproduction. New virus particles are released, either by destroying their host cell or by forming small buds that break off and infect other cells. By cloaking itself in normal cell reproduction, this insidious means of proliferation operates by stealth, escaping detection by the immune system until a critical mass is reached. When the immune system finally catches on, it sends out two kinds of white blood cells: T-lymphocytes (from the thymus) that kill virus infected cells, and B-lymphocytes (from bone marrow) that make antibodies to the virus.

Only the immune system can dispose of viruses. Drugs cannot help. Antibiotics are powerless against these cellular invaders. Sometimes, however, viruses can weaken the immune system so much that it also becomes vulnerable to bacterial invasion. In such cases, antibiotics can clear up the secondary bacterial infections but can do nothing for the original viral infestations.

During acute phases of viral infections it is important to rest, so that the body can devote its energies to immune building. It is also wise to abstain from eating solid foods and to consume only clear liquids (e.g., broths, herbal teas, dilute fruit juices, etc.). At these times one will not usually be hungry anyway. The body needs a break from digesting solid food so that it can devote more attention to detoxifying and building antibodies. The popular saying, "Feed a cold and starve a fever", is a misunderstanding. The original adage was, "If you feed a cold today you will have to starve a fever tomorrow." Feeding the cold short circuits immune processes.

The liver is the chemical factory of the body, which during crises needs to give its primary attention to empowering the immune system. Eating during these times requires the liver to divert time and effort into digestive activity that could be counterproductive during an immune battle. Better to rest, drink plenty of fluids (e.g., water, juices, herbal teas, clear broths), and eat solid food only when genuinely hungry.

Hypoglycemia also makes one susceptible to viral infections. This fact was demonstrated in 1949 when residents of North Carolina reduced their sugar intake by 90 percent, and polio decreased in that state by the same amount. Fluctuating levels of blood sugar create a state of hypoxemia (low oxygen) in tissues, making them vulnerable to invasion by viruses. Eliminating sugar (and all foods with a high glycemic index) enables the immune system to get stronger, empowering it to control viral invaders.

THE COMMON COLD

There can never be a cure for the common cold, because the cold is *not* a disease. It is an eliminative process by which the body disposes of the casualties of its immune battle with viruses, in the mucus and phlegm that is being discharged. Cold symptoms are the evidence that your T- and B-lymphocytes are coming out ahead. Your job is to rest and let them do their thing.

Colds are self-limiting. Drugs can do nothing to speed the process along. It is all up to your immune system – the reason for the tongue-in-cheek remark, "If you have a cold and do nothing it will be gone in a week. If you go to your doctor, it will be gone in seven days."

Some people seem to catch every cold and flu "bug" that goes around and others never seem to catch anything. The former tend to be people with hidden food allergies/sensitivities. There is an obscure adage that says, "You don't catch colds, you eat them." What this means is that if you constantly eat foods to which your body is sensitive, your body's immune system will be so exhausted from having to deal with the daily allergens that it will not be able to muster its resources to ward off other invaders. My body is a case in point. For the first 30 years of my life, I suffered from repeated bouts of colds, flu, laryngitis, pharyngitis, bronchitis, and pneumonia. Whatever was going around, I caught. Since eliminating lactose and gluten (my particular poisons) in 1975, I haven't had a single cold.

THE FLU

Influenza (the "flu") is a self-limiting viral condition that can last up to seven days. Its symptoms can include respiratory infection, fever, chills, headache, back pain, muscle pain, nasal inflammation, coughs, and sore throat. During flu epidemics, those who carry the virus but have no symptoms outnumber those who succumb. Many have immune systems strong enough to keep the virus in check.

Flu vaccines containing the inactivated virus are believed to reduce the incidence rate. The theory is that the immune system recognizes the inactive virus as an invader and creates antibodies to it before its active form has a chance to invade bodily cells. The immunity offered by flu vaccines is not permanent, however. If injecting an inactive virus does not create permanent immunity, then clearly it is not working. Why would it work? If a virus has been inactivated, then it cannot do any harm and thus poses no threat to the immune system.

Even if vaccination with an inactivated virus were capable of mobilizing the desired immune response, its use would still be questionable. Vulnerability to the flu is caused by immune weakness. Those with strong immune systems have no need for the vaccine. Those with weak immune systems could contract the flu from the vaccine.

Flu vaccines have the undeserved reputation of being effective because the overwhelming majority of people who take them were never going to succumb to the flu anyway. The fact that one event [*the flu shot*] precedes another [*not getting sick*] does **not** prove cause and effect.

HERPES

About 30 percent of western populations may suffer periodically from various forms of *Herpes* infections. The most common of these are cold sores (*Herpes simplex*), shingles (*Herpes zoster*), and Epstein-Barr virus.

Cold sores (fever blisters) are tiny, fluid filled blisters that form on and around the lips. They can take up to two weeks to run their natural course before they go away on their own.

Shingles may be caused by leftover chickenpox virus that has remained dormant in nerves since childhood and flares up whenever immune competency is threatened by stress, or by taking corticosteroid drugs or chemotherapy. Symptoms usually manifest as inflammation of nerves (neuritis) and rashes in the face, neck, and upper torso.

Chronic immune challenges, such as a long battle with hidden food allergies, can make one vulnerable to the Epstein-Barr virus – the number one symptom of which is chronic fatigue. Epstein-Barr weakens the immune system even further, making one susceptible to infectious mononucleosis (a bacterial condition).

LYMPHOCYTE PRODUCTION

Lymphocytes provide the body with immune protection from viruses, bacteria, and mutated cells. The thymus gland produces T-lymphocytes (T-cells), which are sent to the spleen and lymph nodes, where they multiply. The thymus also produces thymosin, a hormone that (a) promotes the growth and activity of T-cells after they have left the thymus, and (b) stimulates the spleen and lymph nodes to produce more lymphocytes from their own plasma cells. An adrenal hormone, cortisol, stimulates both the thymus and the lymph nodes. Thus, the three endocrine glands directly involved in lymphocyte protection are the thymus, spleen, and adrenals. Anything which keeps these three glands healthy is of direct benefit to the immune system.

IMMUNE SUPPORT

The nutritional approach to viral infections is to strengthen the body's natural immunity against them – by taking **vitamin C**, **vitamin A**, **glandular concentrates** (thymus, spleen, adrenal), *L. acidophilus* (or similar probiotic), and **L-lysine** (for herpes infections). Also, **oil of oregano** has strong antiviral properties: two drops under the tongue three times daily can produce amazing results.

Vitamin C is the number one nutrient required by the body during immune challenges. Most viral conditions improve significantly from taking 3,000 mg. daily, in divided amounts with meals. Severe challenges may require taking vitamin C to bowel tolerance. This means testing how much vitamin C in a day it takes to produce loose stools or excessive flatulence, then backing off by one third (e.g., if 7,500 mg. of C causes digestive distress, then 5,000 mg. is the optimal daily level to take).

Vitamin A is the number two nutrient the body needs during immune challenges. For adults, 20,000 IU per day is required.

Thymus, spleen, and **adrenal** concentrates – 50 mg. per day of each – provide immune support not possible by any other means. Glandular concentrates from animals provide specific intrinsic cellular factors as nutrients for the same organs in humans. Like cells nourish like cells.

L-lysine – from 1,000 to 3,000 mg. daily – can be helpful in clearing up some viral infections. This amino acid is most efficiently utilized if taken in divided amounts between meals.

THE UNDERDIAGNOSED CONDITION

During his research career, Broda Barnes (PhD, MD) removed the thyroid glands from animals and took detailed notes of the symptoms that this surgery produced. When he became a practising physician, Dr. Barnes observed these same symptoms in many of his patients whose thyroid blood tests were completely normal. The level of thyroid hormones circulating in the blood is an unreliable indicator of how many cells in the body may or may not be receiving enough thyroid hormone for healthy functioning. The blood level of thyroid stimulating hormone (TSH) is also unreliable; many people with low thyroid function (hypothyroidism) have normal blood levels of TSH.

Daily thyroid hormone production is less than 0.001 of an ounce, yet it profoundly affects all of our bodily cells. Thyroxine (T4) is the primary hormone secreted by the thyroid gland. It regulates the rate of metabolism and affects almost all tissues of the body. Thyroxine itself is physiologically inactive, however. It has to be converted into its active form, triiodothyronine (T3) before it can exert its effects. Although some T3 is produced by the thyroid gland, most is converted from T4 by the action of deiodinase enzymes found in many bodily tissues. T3 helps to regulate growth, electrolyte balance, oxidative metabolism, differentiation during cell growth, carbohydrate metabolism, protein metabolism, oxygen consumption, the breakdown of fat, fertility and – most important of all – basal metabolic rate, the speed at which all biochemical reactions take place in the body.

Chronic low thyroid function (hypothyroidism) is rampant. It is the most medically underdiagnosed of all conditions, because blood tests for it are unreliable. Most people with hypothyroidism have normal levels of T4 circulating in their bloodstream; however, their bodies do not convert enough of this hormone to T3, the form in which bodily cells require it.

The thyroid is a gatekeeper. If its hormones function at sub-optimal levels, then nothing else in the body tends to work well either. Hypothyroidism leaves the body vulnerable to allergies, arthritis, asthma, atherosclerosis, autoimmune disorders, breast disease (benign), cancer, cellulitis, chronic fatigue, diabetes, eczema, elevated cholesterol, hypoglycemia, infertility, menstrual disorders, obesity, premature aging, premenstrual syndrome, and sexual dysfunction.

Symptoms of low thyroid function can include:

- not feeling that I have a life of my own.
- not getting to do what I want to do.
- "go to pieces" easily, cry easily.
- muscles stiff in morning, need to limber up.
- fail to feel rested, even after sleeping long hours.
- feel "creaky" after sitting still for some time.
- nauseated in morning.
- start slow in morning, gain speed in afternoon.
- motion sickness when travelling.
- dizzy in morning, or when moving up and down.
- cold hands or feet.
- sensitive to cold, prefer warm climate.
- hair scanty, dry, brittle, dull, lustreless, lifeless.
- hair loss from outer third of eyebrow.
- flaky, dry, rough skin.
- sleeplessness, restlessness, sleep disturbances.
- poor short term memory, forgetfulness.
- poor response to exercising.
- high cholesterol, cholesterol deposits on eyelids.
- constipation, less than one bowel movement daily.
- dislike working under pressure, dislike being watched.
- diminished sex drive, lack of sexual desire.
- gain weight easily, fail to lose on diets.
- difficulty concentrating, easily distracted.
- yellowish tint to skin on hands or feet.
- cracks in bottom of heels.
- clogged sinuses.
- low pulse rate.

- [ ] low body temperature, especially at bed rest.
- [ ] puffiness of face or eyes.
- [ ] swelling of hands or ankles.
- [ ] lumpy breasts, cystic breasts.
- [ ] menstrual irregularity, excess flow, PMS.
- [ ] worse at night: coughing, hoarseness, muscle cramps.

There are two states of functioning that the thyroid gland seeks to maintain – and to switch between, as needed. One is the productivity mode that permits full metabolic functioning at optimal levels. The other is the conservation mode, used for healing and restoration. During acute illness or traumatic injury, the body switches from productivity to conservation, in order to devote its resources to the recovery process. In the conservation mode one craves rest and has no desire for strenuous activity. Body temperature drops, blood pressure may also, and all metabolic activities slow down. A soon as recovery is complete, the thyroid is supposed to switch back into productivity mode. Sometimes, however, it does not – turning what should have been only a temporary adjustment period into a chronic, lasting condition. Many cases of hypothyroidism are thus triggered by disease, injury or some traumatic event. Hypothyroidism is also linked to brain activity. If the brain does not get an adequate supply of glucose (as in hypoglycemia), the thyroid may shift into conservation mode to protect this important organ.

Low thyroid function is also linked to low adrenal function. The thyroid slows down in order not to overstimulate exhausted adrenals. Supporting the adrenals is sometimes all that is needed to restore thyroid function.

A simple home test (for basal temperature) is far more reliable than blood tests for detecting hypothyroidism. This is because it measures a direct effect of thyroid activity – body temperature. Blood tests take only an indirect measure – the amount of thyroid hormone in the blood, which may have little to do with the quantity of hormone that actually reaches the cells that need it.

BASAL TEMPERATURE TEST (BTT)

The basal temperature test (BTT) requires you to take your underarm (axillary) temperature first thing in the morning, before arising, when the body is at complete rest. Men, pre-pubescent and post-menopausal women can take this test at any time. Menstruating women need to do the BTT on the second and third mornings after their flow starts.

To do the BTT, place a liquid-type clinical thermometer, well-shaken down, by the bedside upon retiring. Immediately upon awakening and before stirring from bed, place the bulb of the thermometer under the armpit and hold it there for 10 minutes. Record the reading on two consecutive days. A range of from 36.6 to 36.8 °C (97.8 to 98.2 °F) suggests normal thyroid function. Temperatures below 36.6 °C (97.8 °F) indicate hypothyroidism. Those above 36.8 °C (98.2 °F) indicate an overactive thyroid (hyperthyroidism). In the absence of starving or fasting (which reduce body temperature) and acute fever (which raises it), the BTT is the most reliable means of finding thyroid dysfunction.

For small children who are unable to remain still for 10 minutes, the BTT can be done by taking their rectal temperature for two minutes. Normal rectal temperature is from 37.1°C (98.8°F) to 37.3°C (99.2°F).

Hypothyroidism is so prevalent and its effects so far reaching that anyone with any chronic health problem would do well to take the BTT. If low thyroid function is a causative factor in any condition, that condition does not improve significantly until the thyroid is able to resume its normal functioning.

DAILY TEMPERATURE READINGS

There is a second temperature test that is almost as reliable as the BTT and can be performed any time of day. It simply involves taking one's temperature by mouth four or more times during the day, recording the readings, and calculating a daily average. This average should be 37°C (98.6°F) – or slightly higher for women during times of ovulation.

Body temperature follows a natural daily cycle. It may drop slightly during the evening, a little more during sleep, and gradually increase after waking up and moving around. Ideally, body temperature should be 37°C (or slightly above) between the hours of 10 AM and 5 PM. A daily average below 37°C indicates low thyroid function. Taking multiple daily readings helps one both to discover patterns and to take corrective action more quickly. **Example:** suppose that every day at 4 PM – four hours after eating – you experience an energy "crash" and have to lie down. If every day at 4 PM your body temperature also dropped by, say, one third of a degree, this evidence suggests that thyroid activity slows down when blood sugar is low. Have a mid-afternoon snack to see if it restores both energy and temperature.

RESTORATION

Thyroid support: The following daily quantities of supplementary nutrients enables an otherwise healthy thyroid gland to shift from conversation mode back into full productivity mode. Iodine and tyrosine enable the thyroid gland to produce T4. Selenium and cysteine support the conversion of T4 into T3: **Iodine** (4,000 mcg), **L-tyrosine** (300 mg.), **Selenium** (200 mcg.), and **L-cysteine** (500 mg.). This combo is best taken in divided amounts between meals.

If the thyroid gland has been irradiated, then vital thyroid tissue will have been destroyed and the gland may never recover. The above formula will still be of benefit, however, because of its ability to help the body convert external T4 hormone into T3, the form that cells can actually use. This conversion takes place outside the thyroid gland, in various bodily tissues.

Note 1: Do whatever you need to do to keep your body temperature consistently at 37°C (98.6°F) between the hours of 10 AM and 5 PM, even if it means taking prescription thyroid hormones in addition to the above nutritional formula. (The most natural of these prescription hormones is the generic one called "dessicated thyroid".)

Note 2: Thyroid function usually cannot be restored if adrenal function is weak. This is nature's way of protecting overworked adrenals – by trying to keep the body in conservation mode to give the adrenals some much needed healing time. Sometimes all that is necessary to restore thyroid function is to support the adrenals: in these cases, when the adrenals become rested and well nourished, the thyroid automatically restores itself.

ADRENAL EXHAUSTION

The adrenal glands are two busy little hormone factories that sit atop the kidneys. They produce epinephrine (adrenaline), norepinephrine (noradrenaline), dopamine, glucocorticoids (cortisol, cortisone, corticosterone), mineralcorticoids (aldosterone, dehydroepiandrosterone), and sex hormones (androgens, estrogens, progestins). This spectrum of hormones regulates "fight or flight" reactions to emergency situations, bodily responses to stress, maintenance of carbohydrate reserves, conversion of storage carbohydrate (glycogen) into blood sugar (glucose), blood pressure, electrolyte balance, fluid pressures, kidney function, secondary sexual characteristics and many other functions.

In western society, the adrenals are often overworked and undernourished. Adrenal exhaustion makes the body vulnerable to chronic fatigue, hypoglycemia, allergies, asthma, diabetes, low resistance to infection, low blood pressure, nausea, arthritis, dizziness, poor appetite, weight loss, nervousness and insomnia

Factors that can overtax the adrenals include smoking, narcotics, excess dietary sugars, caffeine, alcohol, stress, and intense emotional reactions. Anxiety, fear, anger, defeatism, feelings of being overpowered, not caring for oneself, and being angry at oneself may be taken in stride if experienced only occasionally. If, however, these feelings become chronic and ingrained, they place the body into a constant "fight or flight" mode that places excess demands on the adrenals.

Common sense suggests that if the adrenals are exhausted, what one needs above all is *rest* to give them time to recuperate. Reduce nutritional and external stressors, work less, do less, and take some quiet time to yourself each day. Simple advice, but to follow it requires breaking deeply ingrained patterns. In most cases the adrenals became exhausted because of a lifelong pattern of continually pushing one's body to its limits – by placing a higher priority on tasks and deadlines, or on other people's needs than on one's own health.

Symptoms of adrenal exhaustion can include:

- ☐ feeling overwhelmed and powerless.
- ☐ eyes sensitive to bright lights, headlights, sunlight.
- ☐ tightness or "lump" in throat, hurts under stress.
- ☐ inability to cope with stressful events.
- ☐ form gooseflesh easily or "cold sweats."
- ☐ voice rises to high pitch or is "lost" during stress.
- ☐ easily shaken up or startled from unexpected noise.
- ☐ prefer being alone, uneasy when centre of attention.
- ☐ blood pressure fluctuates, sometimes too low.
- ☐ perfectionist, set high standards.
- ☐ avoid complaints, try to ignore inconveniences.
- ☐ work off worries, things left undone cause concern.
- ☐ allergies (e.g., skin rash, hay fever, asthma, etc.).
- ☐ mood swings, tendency to cry easily.
- ☐ unusual craving for salt.
- ☐ perspire excessively, sweating of hands or feet.
- ☐ more than usual neck, head, shoulder tension.
- ☐ blood pressure decreases when standing up.

MENOPAUSE

Menopause denotes the cessation of menstruation. In those rare women who have strong adrenal glands and a healthy liver, there are no symptoms – just a smooth transition. As the ovaries stop secreting their sex hormones, the adrenal glands start producing alternate hormones that preserve the secondary feminine characteristics. The vast majority of women, however, have overworked their adrenal glands for decades with stress, caffeine, sugar and/or alcohol – so their transition is anything but smooth, producing the hot flashes and emotional symptoms usually associated with menopause. The above adrenal support prepares the body for menopause and eases the transition.

CHRONIC FATIGUE

Fatigue that never goes away is the symptom of a body upon which demands are continually being made beyond its ability to cope. The adrenal glands have become completely exhausted, and the thyroid slows down in order not to push the adrenals beyond their limits.

During times of overwhelming stress, the thyroid gland shifts into low gear, so to speak, in order to devote the body's resources to healing and recovery. Exercise and activity become very difficult because the body's top priority is to rest. Unfortunately, during this time of needed energy conservation, many people continue to push their bodies to keep up with their hectic lifestyles – thus prolonging what would otherwise have been only a temporary period of adjustment.

The adrenals have become exhausted from a low grade internal battle that is going on all the time. Most usually this is from an immune system that is under siege – from hidden food allergies/intolerances, a candida/ yeast infection, Epstein-Barr virus, mononucleosis – or from a leaky gut that causes the body to work overtime producing IgG antibodies to neutralize the foreign protein molecules that get into the blood. Identify and overcome the immune challenges. Nourish and support the adrenals and thyroid.

ADRENAL SUPPORT

Daily amounts of nutrients that support adrenal function include **vitamin C** (2,000 mg.), **pantothenic acid** (up to 1,500 mg.), and **vitamin B-12** (1,000 mcg.) – best taken at the same time, in divided amounts with meals. During times of acute stress, depression or grief, the adrenal glands' need for vitamin C soars. In such cases it is often beneficial to take vitamin C to bowel tolerance. This means finding out how much vitamin C it takes to cause either loose stools or excess flatulence, then backing off by one-third. [Example: *If it takes 9,000 mg. of vitamin C to stress the bowels, then 6,000 mg. is the optimal daily amount to take.*]

THE CHOLESTEROL MYTH

If you believe that normal cholesterol levels protect you from heart attacks, you could be dead wrong – literally. No matter how carefully you follow a low-cholesterol diet and no matter how much butter or how many eggs you avoid, your chances of dying prematurely from a heart attack are about the same as if you had *not* restricted your cholesterol intake.

The cholesterol-as-cause theory is pseudoscientific nonsense. Cholesterol is a major component of the plaque that occludes arteries; however, cholesterol is a later constituent that is laid down in the plaque, not the first. Cholesterol is a slippery, waxy substance that cannot possibly adhere to a smooth, healthy arterial lining.

There is just as much cholesterol circulating in our veins as in our arteries, but plaque is found only in arteries and never in veins. If cholesterol were the cause of circulatory impairment, then why does it not occlude veins?

Epidemiological evidence gives no credence to the cholesterol myth. The first heart attack documented in medical records occurred in 1910. For more than a century prior to that time, the typical western diet, especially in rural areas, included large quantities of eggs, butter, lard, bacon, sausage, pork, and red meat – and there were zero deaths from heart disease.

The cholesterol scare has caused many people to stop consuming eggs. That's too bad, because eggs are the most nourishing food we can eat. They provide the highest quality protein of all, plus all minerals and vitamins (except C). The reason there is no vitamin C in eggs is because chickens have no need for it. Their livers produce all that they need.

BENEFITS OF CHOLESTEROL

Cholesterol is a vital substance found in every cell in the body. Cholesterol is made by the liver and distributed throughout the body, where it converts sunlight under the skin into vitamin D (cholecalciferol), becomes a constituent of bile acids (for digesting fats), and participates in the structure of cellular membranes. Cholesterol is part of the myelin sheath that insulates nerve cells. Seventeen percent of brain tissue is cholesterol. Cholesterol is also used to produce sex hormones (estrogen, testosterone, progesterone) and adrenal hormones (cortisol, aldosterone).

Cholesterol is so important that the less of it we eat, the more our bodies produce. For those on omnivorous diets, the liver produces about 80 per cent of the cholesterol the body needs, with only 20 percent coming from food sources. Since cholesterol is found only in animal foods, on a total vegetarian (vegan) diet, 100 per cent of bodily cholesterol is produced by the body itself. High blood cholesterol levels (hypercholesterolemia) have little or nothing to do with the amount of cholesterol consumed.

There is no direct correlation between serum cholesterol levels and the incidence of coronary artery disease. Reports suggest that up to 80 percent of those who have heart attacks or bypass surgery have cholesterol levels within normal range.

The cholesterol found in arterial plaque may actually be there in a protective role, as an antioxidant of last resort – when the body lacks sufficient dietary antioxidants (e.g., vitamin C, vitamin E, selenium). In this role, cholesterol covers over arterial patches and gives up electrons (i.e., becomes oxidized) in order to neutralize free radicals and prevent further damage to the arteries.

MISUSE OF SCIENCE

In 1915, Nikolai Anitschkow fed cholesterol to rabbits and observed that various tissues throughout their bodies became saturated with cholesterol. The cholesterol in the rabbits' arteries, however, bore no resemblance to the foam cells found in human arteries. No surprise here. Rabbits are herbivores (total vegetarians) that do not have a digestive system capable of breaking down or assimilating cholesterol, which is found only in foods of animal origin. If Anitschkow had used omnivores (e.g., rats, monkeys) as subjects, his results would have been very different.

In 1953, Ancel Keys published a report showing a supposed correlation between the consumption of fats/cholesterol and the incidence of heart disease in six countries. Mr. Keys committed selection bias, however, because he had data from 22 countries but chose only those six which supported his preconceived notion. One of the countries he excluded was France, which has both a high consumption of fat and a low incidence of heart disease. Had Keys plotted all 22 sets of data, there would have been no correlation whatsoever, simply random points on a graph.

Keys may have been the first researcher to manipulate statistics, but he was not the last. All of the studies allegedly implicating cholesterol as the cause for heart disease are based on either flawed research or results which are statistically insignificant.

In statistical analysis, there is something called the "coefficient of correlation", which is designated by an "r". This variable measures how close your results came to your prediction. If $r = 1.0$, this means that your theory predicted 100 percent of the observations made during your study. If $r = 0.0$, this means that your theory has absolutely no relationship to the real world. If $r = 0.5$, this is equivalent to a coin toss: on average you are right half of the time. Now, are you sitting down for this? The highest (yes, the highest) coefficient of correlation published in any cholesterol study was 0.30 – worse than flipping a coin.

CHOLESTEROL LOWERING DRUGS

Cholesterol lowering drugs are potentially lethal. They reduce cholesterol everywhere in the body, including in the brain – where cholesterol acts as an insulator to prevent water from entering nerve cells and shorting out electrical circuits. Evidence shows that taking cholesterol lowering drugs increases one's risk of dying from suicide or violent accident. These drugs cause momentary brain lapses, which are most unfortunate if they happen when one is pulling out into heavy traffic.

Cholesterol lowering drugs also interfere with the body's production of coenzyme Q_{10} – a natural antioxidant found in every cell in the body. Anyone who insists on taking these drugs needs to take supplementary CoQ_{10}.

Cholesterol lowering drugs may actually contribute to atherosclerosis by depleting the natural antioxidant CoQ_{10} that is normally present in arterial cells. There is no direct relationship between cholesterol levels and atherosclerosis. Someone with zero or minimal arterial damage who takes drugs to lower cholesterol could actually be accelerating the formation of plaque in their arteries.

NORMALIZING CHOLESTEROL LEVELS

The misplaced focus on dietary cholesterol has diverted attention away from other important evidence: both cholesterol and triglyceride levels tend to rise in response to dietary sugars, caffeine and alcohol. Often serum cholesterol can be normalized by the complete elimination of concentrated sweets (e.g., sugar, candy, pastries, cookies, soda pop, etc.), caffeine (e.g., coffee, tea, colas) and alcoholic beverages.

If you have concerns about elevated cholesterol levels or unfavorable ratios, try this four part program: (1) eliminate dietary sugars, (2) increase dietary fiber, (3) drink more water, and (4) get more exercise. If after three weeks there has been no significant improvement, then do a basal temperature test (BTT) to see if your thyroid gland is sluggish. Elevated cholesterol can be an overlooked symptom of hypothyroidism.

If all else fails, there is a cholesterol normalizing combo that users claim is more effective than prescription drugs and has no side effects. It includes the following daily amounts: **Red Yeast Rice extract** (400 mg.), **Guggul Resin extract** (300 mg.), and **Niacin** (100 mg.) – all of which are best taken at the same times, in divided amounts with meals. Niacin tends to produce a natural flushing response that makes the skin temporarily reddish and itchy. If you find this uncomfortable, reduce the total daily amount of niacin to 50 mg.

<u>Note</u>: *When you are successful at bringing your cholesterol levels into line, you will have done nothing to reduce your risk of having a heart attack or stroke. Most cardiovascular accidents occur in those whose cholesterol levels are within normal range.*

FREE RADICAL DAMAGE

Free radicals are highly reactive molecular fragments that interact rapidly and aggressively with other molecules in the body to create abnormal cells. They can penetrate into the DNA of a cell and change its "blueprint" so that it now produces renegade cells that proliferate out of control.

Free radicals are unstable. They have unpaired electrons in their outer orbits, which cause them to react almost instantly with any substance in their vicinity. Oxygen free radicals are especially dangerous because they react readily with many other molecules. They are the reason we need antioxidants, agents that protect cells from the damaging effects of peroxides and superoxide (highly reactive forms of oxygen).

The body uses free radicals, in a controlled way, to kill invading bacteria and virus-infected cells, to neutralize other free radicals, and to detoxify harmful chemicals. Outside this regulated environment, however, free radicals destroy cellular membranes, enzymes, genetic material and even life itself. They accelerate aging and contribute to the development of atherosclerosis, cancer, and cataracts. They damage collagen by causing a cross-linkage of molecules and the loss of elasticity. Wrinkled skin, stiff joints, high blood pressure and premature aging are often the result of this process of deterioration.

Free radicals are released in the body from overexposure to sunlight –from the breaking down or detoxification of many chemical compounds, such as petrochemicals (e.g., in drugs, artificial food colorings, smog), preservatives in processed meats (nitrates, nitrites), exhaust fumes (carbon monoxide), cleaning fluids (carbon tetrachloride), the tar in tobacco smoke – from drinking or swimming in chlorinated water (which forms chloroform in the body) – from cadmium and other heavy metals – from radiation (X-rays, gamma radiation, cosmic radiation, microwaves, cell phones) – and from rancid and adulterated fats. The more we expose ourselves to free radicals, the less capable our immune systems are of protecting us from their damage.

Some common food substances contribute to excess free radical production. These include polyunsaturated oils, alcohol, and sugar. Studies suggest that both oxidative damage and free radical production may be linked to spikes in sugar consumption. This may be why diabetics are at high risk for atherosclerosis: arteries are continually flooded with excess glucose (blood sugar).

One free radical hazard is internally generated. During constipation, renegade disease-causing chemicals are released into the colon and the bloodstream. Our ancestors ate unprocessed foods, rich in fiber, which tend to fill out the colon and aid in its evacuation – the way nature intended. We would do well to emulate their habits. Because the fiber has been removed from refined flour and sugar products, these foods tend to be constipating.

Stress and overwork also increase our risk of free radical damage. Whether the stress itself creates free radicals, or whether it prevents our immune processes from neutralizing free radicals is unknown. Either way, the result is the same. Anything you can do to relieve stress reduces your body's risk of free radical damage. Balance work with pleasure, take daily rest breaks, exercise regularly, be spontaneous, socialize, and do something every day just for fun.

FATS AND OILS

Polyunsaturated oils are chemically unstable. That is because they have a number of loose, double carbon bonds in their molecular structure. When subjected to heat or air, they oxidize rapidly to form harmful free radicals. The more unsaturated the oil, the more potentially hazardous it is. Examples of oils that are predominately polyunsaturated are safflower, sunflower, corn, soy, wheat germ, walnut, flax, pumpkin and cottonseed.

The most hazardous vegetable oils are the ones used in restaurants for deep frying. Those oils are heated and re-heated many times over. They are rancid, but you cannot taste or smell that rancidity because of deodorants that manufacturers add.

Other hazardous vegetable oils are those which have been hydrogenated to form margarine, shortening and other manufactured or tinkered fats. These substances are food artefacts rather than actual foods. They contain peroxidized fats, *trans* fatty acids and other modified fat molecules which can compromise immune processes.

Even the highly promoted cold pressed oils can be harmful. Many of them are processed at a "cold" temperature of over 200 °F (generated by the friction of the machinery). As soon as they are exposed to air they deteriorate rapidly – and if used in cooking their destruction is virtually guaranteed.

Healthy fatty acids are critical to our survival. They form part of the membranes that surround every cell in the body. They help protect against degenerative diseases. They are precursors to the hormone-like prostaglandins that regulate gastric secretions, pancreatic functions and the release of pituitary hormones. Fatty acids combine with glycerol to form triglycerides, which act as carriers for vitamins A, D and E – and also help to convert beta carotene into vitamin A.

Fatty acids are of three basic types: saturated (e.g., palmitic acid, stearic acid), monounsaturated (e.g., oleic acid) and polyunsaturated (e.g., linoleic, linolenic, arachidonic). All of the fats and oils in our diet consist of various combinations and proportions of these three groups. If our diets provide an adequate supply of all the basic fatty acids, our bodies can pick and choose the best ones for the tasks that need to be accomplished on any given day. If the best ones are not available, then we force our bodies to make do with substitutes. Unfortunately, if only rancid or per-oxidized fats or *trans* fatty acids are provided, then we end up with inferior cellular membranes, plus inadequate prostaglandins and an overloaded immune system which struggles in vain to stave off free radical damage.

Two fatty acids are critical. They are called "essential" because we need them for survival but our bodies cannot make them. We have to get them from food. They are linoleic acid (omega-6) and linolenic acid (omega-3). Without these essential fatty acids we perish. With enough of them (and in the presence of adequate vitamins and minerals), the body can make all of the other fatty acids it needs.

The essential fatty acids we need are found in high proportions in those oils that are predominately polyunsaturated. However, these are the very oils that are most prone to deterioration and the production of free radicals. Therefore, balance is required. We need to do without overdoing. Fortunately, those fats and oils that are predominately saturated or monounsaturated also contain smaller but significant amounts of essential fatty acids.

Our primitive ancestors were safe from hazardous oils. They were unable to extract oils from plants. They received all of the essential fatty acids they needed from the natural whole foods that they ate – including poultry fat, animal fat, fish, avocado, egg yolk, olives, butter, nuts, and seeds. There is wisdom in consuming our polyunsaturates as part of the whole nut or seed, where nature's package protects them from deterioration. It is risky to consume them as extracted and refined oils, in unnatural and potentially dangerous proportions.

Nuts and seeds that are heated or roasted lose their natural protection against the potentially harmful breakdown of the polyunsaturates they contain. Be especially wary of roasted nuts that are heavily salted. Their saltiness may hide the taste of rancidity.

Organic flaxseed oil provides approximately 57 percent linolenic acid, 16 percent linoleic acid and 18 percent oleic acid – and is used therapeutically as a partial treatment for a number of degenerative conditions. Raw flaxseed oil, however, is highly susceptible to deterioration that quickly transforms it into an overabundant source of free radicals. A healthier choice is flaxseed oil that has been specially processed at 40 °C in the total absence of oxygen. This particular oil is hermetically sealed into opaque capsules and bottled in the presence of nitrogen into light-resistant bottles, making it resistant to the destructive influences of oxygen, heat, and light.

Both the quality and quantity of fats and oils we consume are critical to our health. If our total fat intake is too low, we compromise cellular immunity and increase our risk of developing cancer. If our total fat intake is too high, the body uses first the fatty acids it can most easily assimilate, leaving the hazardous ones to circulate throughout the lymphatic system where they can cause tissue damage and tumors. Balance is required.

PINCH TEST

Every person, every day, is bombarded by free radicals, from both external hazards and dietary sources. We differ in our ability to withstand free radical damage, however. If you want to know how much your body has already been affected by free radicals, here is a simple test: Extend your hand, palm down, in a relaxed position. Pinch the skin on the back of your hand and lift the fold upwards. Release this fold of skin and see how long it takes to pull back into position. If you are young or have minimal free radical damage, your skin will snap back instantly. Where there is considerable cross-linkage of collagen, the skin fold will slowly slip back into place, sometimes taking several seconds.

RISKS FROM POLYUNSATURATED OILS

Polyunsaturated oils are a mixed blessing. They provide essential fatty acids, but in an unstable form. Each molecule of a polyunsaturated fat contains a number of loose double carbon bonds that readily break apart upon exposure to heat, light, or air – releasing a cascade of free radicals in the body. The more unsaturated an oil is, the greater its risk. Safflower, sunflower, corn, soy, sesame, and canola oils are hazardous when heated – and all of them have been heated during processing at the factory. Even so-called cold pressed oils have been subjected to temperatures of up to 200°F (90°C) from the friction generated by the extraction machinery.

OLIVE OIL TO THE RESCUE

Monounsaturated fatty acids (omega-9) have only one loose double carbon bond in their molecular structure. That makes them much more resistant to deterioration from heat and light than the polyunsaturates. Examples of oils high in monounsaturates are olive, almond, macadamia, avocado, hazelnut/filbert, pecan, and pistachio. Peanut oil is somewhere in the middle – not quite as stable as the preceding oils yet more stable than the polyunsaturates.

Olive oil is about 79 percent oleic acid (monounsaturated), 13 percent saturated fats, and only 8 percent polyunsaturates. Oleic acid contributes stability to cellular membranes, helping them to resist invasion by free radicals. (This may be one reason why Mediterranean diets that include olive oil as a staple are associated with a low incidence of heart disease.) Oleic acid is also the predominant fatty acid in mother's milk – and the predominant fat in sebum, the protective substance secreted by sweat glands.

FREE RADICAL SCAVENGERS

The body produces enzymes which act as free radical scavengers (or inhibitors), whose role is to neutralize free radicals before they cause harm: catalase breaks down hydrogen peroxide, glutathione peroxidase neutralizes other peroxides, and superoxide dismustase (SOD) neutralizes superoxide. To function optimally, these scavenger enzymes require daily supplements that include: **selenium** (250 mcg.), **zinc** (30 mg.), **manganese** (15 mg.), **DL-methionine** (250 mg.), and **L-cysteine** (750 mg.).

ANTIOXIDANTS

Antioxidants are agents that help protect cells from the damaging effects of oxygen free radicals. In addition to its role in supporting scavenger enzymes, selenium is also a powerful antioxidant. Two other antioxidants that are needed to win the war against free radicals are **vitamin C** (4,000 mg. daily), and **vitamin E** (600 I.U. daily).

DIABETES

Diabetes mellitus is a chronic disorder of carbohydrate metabolism characterized by high blood sugar (hyperglycemia) and excess glucose in the urine (glycosuria). Diabetes can occur either when the pancreas does not secrete enough insulin – or when the cells of the body become resistant to insulin, preventing blood sugar (glucose) from entering the cells – in either case leading to serious complications, such as greatly increased risks for heart disease, stroke, gangrene, kidney disease, loss of sight (retinopathy), and loss of nerve function (neuropathy).

Classic symptoms of diabetes include excessive urination, excessive thirst, and excessive appetite. Other symptoms may also be present, such as boils and carbuncles, vascular changes, and a sweet (acetone) odor of the breath.

Diabetes is divided into two major types. Type I, or insulin-dependent diabetes mellitus (IDDM), usually has its onset before the age of 25 and is related to insulin deficiency. It is believed to be an autoimmune disorder that destroys the beta cells of the pancreas (those which secrete insulin) – as if the body has become allergic to its own pancreas cells.

Type II, or non-insulin-dependent diabetes mellitus (NIDDM) is much more common than type I. In type II the pancreas typically overproduces insulin but the cells of the body have become resistant to it. There are a number of factors contributing to cellular resistance to insulin, and one of them may sometimes be allergy to insulin itself. Most cases of type II diabetes can be controlled by diet and supplements.

Complications of diabetes include acidosis due to excess production of ketone bodies, low resistance to infections (especially in the extremities), cardiovascular impairment, kidney disorders; disturbances in electrolyte balance, and toxemia of pregnancy. Diabetics are prone to develop retinopathy, glaucoma, and neuropathy. Cardiovascular disease is the major cause of death in diabetics. In addition, peripheral vascular disease may lead to ischemia (reduced blood flow) and gangrene of the lower limbs.

High levels of insulin are caustic to the arteries, inflaming them and causing injury that produces plaque (atherosclerosis) and stimulates the synthesis of lipids (fats) in the arterial wall. These fats appear to be formed for the purpose of protecting the artery from further injury from the insulin.

When blood sugar is elevated, it produces an increase in the production of free radicals that cause oxidative damage to arteries and capillaries. This excess production of free radicals happens to everyone after eating a high glycemic meal, usually only during the first half hour while blood sugar is rising. If blood sugar is constantly high, however, there is no relief from the onslaught of free radicals.

Excess glucose in the blood also attaches itself to proteins and fats, altering their structures. This process (called "glycation") causes proteins in the inner lining of blood vessels to become sticky and glob together. It also increases the likelihood that bits of arterial plaque may break off and plug an artery, thus causing a stroke or heart attack.

THE DIABETIC DIET

The ideal diet for both forms of diabetes is to eat as few processed foods as possible, to have frequent small meals throughout the day, to increase dietary fiber (e.g., vegetables, whole grains, fresh fruits), to restrict total fat intake, to use mono-unsaturated fats (e.g., olive oil) over other dietary fats, and to avoid all foods with a high glycemic index (i.e., the measure of a food to raise blood glucose).

A diet that is high in fats tends to obstruct the cell's ability to receive glucose, but monounsaturated fats (in moderation) seem to have a protective and normalizing effect on cellular membranes. Thus it wise to consume two tablespoonsful of olive oil daily and to restrict one's intake of other fats.

NUTRITIONAL SUPPORT

There is a combination of supplements that reduces insulin resistance, thus enabling cells to make more efficient use of glucose. This formula is of significant benefit to type II diabetes (non-insulin dependent) – and is also of some help to type I diabetes. The daily amounts of nutrients required are **magnesium** (200 mg.), **trimethylglycine** (300 mg.), **zinc** (30 mg.), **alpha-lipoic acid** (200 mg.), **manganese** (15 mg.), **chromium** (200 mcg.), and **vanadium** (300 mcg.)

Diabetics are the highest risk group for cardiovascular diseases. In addition to the above – and sometimes instead of the above – it is in their best interests to take the arterial cleansing formula (ACF) described in the next chapter, "Unplug the Arteries".

UNPLUG THE ARTERIES

Experience is the only proof.
Everything else is theory.

Cardiovascular diseases have reached epidemic proportions. They kill more people than all other disease causes combined. Every year, 735,000 Americans have a heart attack, of which 325,000 are fatal. Statistically speaking, there is a about a 44 percent chance your first heart attack will kill you.

The good news is that none of these statistics need apply to you or your loved ones. There is an effective and time tested natural way to correct atherosclerosis (arteriosclerosis), the gradual narrowing of arteries which leads to heart attacks, strokes and gangrene. For over 30 years, many thousands of Canadians have been using this safe and simple method to reduce the deposits in their arteries that have been building up over the years. This is prevention at its best – to reverse the cause of the problem before it produces any life-threatening symptoms. Innumerable people have used it to relieve angina and leg pains, to eliminate the need for bypass surgery, and to avoid amputations.

The body has an incredible, innate ability to heal itself – provided we give it the both the raw materials and the conditions it needs to do so. If you give your body everything it needs, it can heal damaged arteries just as easily as it can heal a cut finger.

Expect some surprises. Cholesterol does *not* cause heart disease. The first detectable signs of occluding arteries are *not* fatty streaks. Bypass surgery does *not* extend lives. Polyunsaturated oils may do more harm than good. Will Rogers once said, *"It ain't what we don't know that gives us trouble; it is what we know that ain't so."*

YOU ARE YOUR OWN HEALER

Your body is self-repairing. Heart disease has become a rampant killer only because (a) we expose our bodies to insults at a rate far faster than our natural immune processes can neutralize them, and (b) we do not give our bodies enough of the vital raw materials required to fortify these self-repairing systems. The arterial cleansing program (*aka* "nutritional bypass") answers both of these concerns.

Your body has innate healing wisdom. You can direct the course of your own health without having to trust blindly in anyone else to do it for you. Arterial cleansing gives you the opportunity to improve the quality and perhaps also the length of your life, as it has done and is doing for many thousands of others.

EARLY DETECTION

Atheromatous plaque builds up on arterial walls gradually, over years and decades. Arteries in vulnerable locations progressively become narrower and narrower – until one day they become so constricted as to precipitate a cardiovascular accident, such as a heart attack or stroke. These events happen when a blood clot, undissolved matter (embolus), or a blob of cholesterol gets stuck in a narrowed opening, or when the artery itself seals shut.

Tissue dies when it is suddenly deprived of its blood supply. If the sinoatrial node (pacemaker) of the heart is affected, then that heart attack is necessarily fatal. If other parts of the heart are affected, there is a good chance that the person will survive, given the proper care. Unless the causative atherosclerotic progression is either halted or reversed, however, subsequent heart attacks and/or strokes are likely. Arteries continue to deteriorate unless and until properly treated with what has been termed, "nutritional arterial cleansing".

Until an artery is about 70 percent blocked there are usually no symptoms. Unfortunately for some people, the first symptom is death. It is not unusual to hear of someone who has suffered a heart attack within hours or days of having been given a clean bill of health. Stress tests and electrocardiograms can find only existing and prior heart problems; they cannot predict when a future heart attack may occur.

EARLY WARNING SIGNS

There are a number of early warning signs which indicate deteriorating circulation. See if any apply to you:

- □ Fingers and/or toes often go cold
- □ Arms and/or legs often "go to sleep"
- □ Numbness or heaviness in arms or legs
- □ Cramps in hand when writing
- □ Sharp, diagonal crease in earlobe
- □ Tingling sensations in lips or fingers
- □ Short walk causes cramping or pains in the legs
- □ Memory not as good as it used to be
- □ Ankles swell late in the day
- □ Breathlessness on slight exertion or on lying down
- □ Whitish ring under outer part of cornea in the eye
- □ High blood pressure
- □ Chest pain after physical exercise or emotional stress

If you experience several of the above – or if you experience only one of these symptoms intensely – your circulatory system is crying out for attention.

One of the items on the above list is a sharp diagonal crease in the earlobe. This is an interesting phenomenon. It is caused by the earlobe's folding in on itself from sleeping on one's side. After the arteries have been cleared of plaque, however, the blood supply is never restored to the earlobe. Its crease remains permanent. It seems that body has more important priorities for improved circulation than to bother with a cosmetic appendage.

MEASURING ARTERIAL BLOCKAGES

Coronary angiogram (arteriogram): the most popular coronary diagnostic tool for several decades. The angiogram is a procedure whereby a radioactive dye is injected into the arteries and a film taken to estimate the degree of blockage. If the angiographer reports a 75 percent occlusion of the left main anterior descending artery, surgery is usually recommended. Angiograms can be hazardous. Death rates of up to one percent have been reported. There is a possibility of a heart attack or stroke during the procedure or even months later. There are also risks of torn arteries, infection, and allergic reaction to the dye.

Doppler ultrasound: a safe, non-invasive diagnostic method for determining blood flow velocity in coronary, carotid and other arteries. Arterial blockages can actually be seen on a television monitor, the same way that ultrasound is used to show expectant mothers the developing fetus.

In 1984, a 52-year old man was diagnosed at Sunnybrook Hospital with coronary artery blockages that he saw for himself on the video monitor. After four months on the arterial cleansing formula, the same ultrasound test was repeated at Toronto General Hospital. No arterial blockages could be found. The doctors at TGH "knew" that this was impossible, and so accused the doctors at Sunnybrook of misdiagnosis.

Digital pulse analysis (DPA): an indirect method of estimating arterial health. DPA uses plethysmography to record changes in volume of blood flow and also grades arterial flexibility. The less flexible the arteries, the more plaque is inferred to have accumulated. DPA can be applied in an office setting rather than a hospital. It can be used (a) to indicate the need for arterial cleansing, and (b) to chart one's progress using the arterial cleansing formula (ACF).

Symptom amelioration: any symptom that can be quantified is a reliable indicator of progress using the ACF. For example, if you could walk only 10 yards before experiencing leg pains and after one month on the ACF you can walk 200 yards without pain, there clearly has been a reduction in arterial blockages. Similarly, if you used to have angina daily and now you never get it, there has been a reduction of at least one coronary artery blockage.

Endoscopic photography: a procedure that involves snaking a tube and optical system into an artery and taking a picture. On the following page are before-and-after photos sent to me by a doctor in Germany. Both photos were taken inside the same coronary artery of the same 68-year old man. The upper photo was taken prior to treatment. The lower was taken after five months on the Arterial cleansing formula. (Optimal arterial cleansing in a 68-year old man usually takes about seven months.)

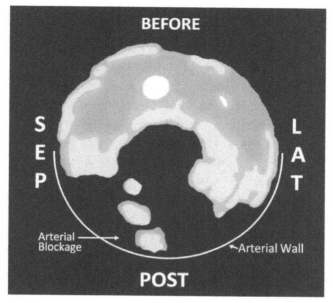

Before: This is an interior photo of a coronary artery in a 68-year old male patient, prior to treatment.

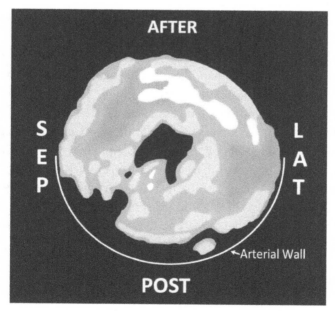

After: This is an interior photo of the same coronary artery in the same 68-year old male patient, after five months of nutritional therapy. This therapy consisted of taking 10 tablets per day of a broad spectrum arterial cleansing formula that includes 16 vitamins, 9 minerals, 2 amino acids and 3 glandular concentrates.

DIABETIC COMPLICATIONS

Anyone with diabetes mellitus is at high risk for cardiovascular accidents. According to the American Heart Association, from 65 to 75 percent of diabetics may die from heart attacks, strokes or ruptured aneurysms. In addition, diabetics are plagued with impaired peripheral circulation that causes kidney damage (nephropathy), blindness from retinopathy, and amputations of gangrenous toes, feet, or legs. High levels of glucose and insulin in the blood accelerate the development of atherosclerosis, carrying circulatory impairment to extremes.

It is commonly accepted that high levels of insulin are caustic to the interior wall of arteries, aging them and causing injury that produces plaque. Excess insulin inflames (i.e., damages) arteries and stimulates the synthesis of lipids (fats) in the arterial wall. These fats appear to be formed for purpose of protecting the artery from further injury from the insulin.

When blood sugar is elevated, it produces an increase in the production of the free radicals that can cause oxidative damage to arteries and capillaries. This excess production of free radicals happens to everyone after eating a high glycemic meal, usually during only the first half hour while blood sugar is rising. If blood sugar is constantly high, however, there is no relief from the onslaught of free radicals.

Excess glucose in the blood also attaches itself to proteins and fats, altering their structures. This process is referred to as "glycation", which *Wikipedia* defines as "the result of co-valent bonding of a protein or lipid molecule with a sugar molecule, such as glucose." Glycation causes proteins in the inner lining of blood vessels to become sticky and to glob together. It also increases the likelihood that bits of plaque may break off and plug up a blood vessel, thus causing a stroke or heart attack.

The arterial cleansing formula includes **chromium** and **magnesium**, both of which minerals help to regulate blood sugar metabolism. Some diabetics taking the ACF have been able to reduce their bodies' requirements for insulin injections.

BYPASS SURGERY

Coronary artery bypass surgery creates a shunt that permits blood to travel from the aorta to a branch of a blocked coronary artery at a point past the obstruction. Since 1968 bypass surgery has been promoted as a life extending procedure. The evidence suggests otherwise.

In 1983, the National Heart, Lung and Blood Institute released its findings of their 10-year Coronary Artery Surgery Study of 780 participants from 15 different hospitals. Results showed that those who received bypass surgery had no better survival rate than those in similar condition who didn't have this surgery. There was no difference in quality of life between the surgical and non-surgical group. Of those participants selected for surgery, 1.4 percent died during the operation or within 30 days.

A survey at two large military hospitals revealed that 63 percent of patients who underwent coronary bypass surgery before their 36th birthdays either failed to improve, relapsed or died. Of patients aged 45 and over, 45 percent had similarly poor outcomes. [*Medical Abstracts*, Sept/86]

A study of 767 men at several European medical centers showed that survival rates were no better in many patients who have had coronary bypass surgery than in those who received only drug treatment. One hundred and nine who had the surgery died within 12 years (compared to 92 in the control group). Thirty-four bypass patients had a total of 44 repeat operations, and five of those 34 patients died. [*New England Journal of Medicine,* Aug. 11/88]

Bypass surgery performed on the carotid artery is just as questionable. Dr. Henry Barnett, Professor of Neurology at the University of Western Ontario gave a report in Toronto at the July/85 International Congress of Neurologic Surgery. In it he showed, through clinical trial, that carotid bypass surgery (then 20 years old) was worthless. Final analysis of the data showed that patients receiving this surgery had more strokes and fatalities (15 percent) than similar patients in similar condition who didn't receive surgery (four percent strokes and fatalities).

Bypass surgery consists of rerouting blood flow around blockages by grafting in a piece of vein taken from elsewhere in the body. The bypass can be performed only on parts of the body that are accessible to the scalpel – such as the front of the heart, the abdomen, or in the neck. It is impossible to bypass blood vessels on the back of the heart or anywhere in the skull.

Every surgery has risks. The bypass may have an estimated mortality rate from one to four percent on the operating table, and about 20 percent or more within two years. Sometimes blood clots from the operation migrate and lodge themselves in narrowed arteries elsewhere. Side effects from this operation include strokes, personality changes, decreased IQ, vision loss, and depression.

Any relief that the bypass provides is only temporary. This surgery does nothing to stop blockages from reforming at or near the original site. It does nothing to halt progressive deterioration elsewhere in the arterial tree. One bypass operation often leads to a second or even a third some years down the road. And there is a limit. Sooner or later the body runs out of operable sites.

OTHER SURGERIES

Angioplasty is a less invasive surgical alternative to the bypass. A popular version of this technique involves inserting a balloon catheter into an occluded blood vessel, inflating it, and then rubbing it back and forth to expand the artery and compress the plaque. Another version involves reaming out the blockage with a high speed, very fine drill. A report in the *New England Journal of Medicine* (Sept. 22/88) suggests that in 25 to 40 percent of coronary angioplasty cases, the same vessel becomes blocked again – usually within six months after the procedure.

A **stent** is a stainless steel, self-expanding mesh inserted into a coronary artery. It is typically used to prevent blood vessels from re-closing after bypass surgery or angioplasty.

Surgical methods of treating atherosclerosis attempt either to remove plaque or to bypass plugged arteries, after the damage has been done. These surgeries treat effects but are incapable of correcting causes. Unless the atherosclerosis itself is halted, further surgeries are likely to be required.

CHELATION THERAPY

There is a safe and effective medical technique for removing arterial plaque. It consists of injecting a slow drip solution of magnesium disodium EDTA into a vein over a three hour period. It usually takes 30 such treatments (at $100 each) to achieve optimal results. Because EDTA therapy does not correct the cause of the problem, it is wise to repeat this series of injections at regular intervals of every five years or so. Those who take the Arterial cleansing formula immediately after EDTA chelation and stay on it consistently should never have the need for a second round of EDTA treatments.

EDTA (ethylene diamine tetra-acetic acid) is a synthetic amino acid that binds to minerals in the arterial plaque (calcium, iron, copper, lead, mercury) and removes them from the body. (About 40 percent of the dry weight of plaque is comprised of calcium.) EDTA is neither altered nor metabolized by the body. Once it binds to a mineral, it is rapidly filtered out by the kidneys into the urine. The EDTA molecule leaves the body intact, bringing minerals with it. Because EDTA is inert, the body has no need or use for it. Therefore, it cannot be absorbed through the intestinal tract. EDTA works only intravenously.

The word, "chelate", is a chemical term that means to combine with a ring structure, as a claw would grasp an object. Chelation involves the surrounding of mineral or metallic ions by ring structured molecules. The Arterial cleansing formula is sometimes referred to as "oral chelation"; however, this term is only a partial description. Although there are a number of nutrients in the ACF which have chelating effects, this nutritional formula works in a number of interrelated ways, perhaps the most significant of which is to act as a "detergent" that dissolves fats in the arterial plaque.

The natural chelating factors in the ACF include **L-cysteine, DL-methionine**, and **Vitamin C**. There is also **magnesium**, which dissolves calcium deposits – and **vitamin B-1** (thiamine), which facilitates the removal of lead from tissues.

The arterial cleansing formula enables the body to repair underlying damage to the artery walls, by giving the body the raw materials it needs to do its own healing. This is something that EDTA chelation cannot do. Thus, the ACF has the potential to remove more plaque than EDTA therapy can. Some of the plaque has been purposely laid down by the body to patch tears and reinforce weak spots in artery walls. Until those weak areas have been repaired or strengthened nutritionally, the body will <u>not</u> let go of plaque that it needs to maintain structural integrity.

BENEFITS OF ARTERIAL CLEANSING

Amputations avoided. Over the years, many feet and legs have been saved from amputation by taking the arterial cleansing formula (ACF). This is a medical miracle that happens routinely.

Angina Relieved. Angina pectoris is severe pain around the heart caused by a relative deficiency of oxygen supply to the heart. It often occurs after increased activity, exercise, or a stressful event. Pain or numbness may radiate to the left shoulder and down the left arm, or it may radiate to the back or jaw. Angina is caused by blockages in one or more coronary arteries and can be relieved by taking the ACF.

Leg pains gone. Intermittent claudication is a severe pain in the calf muscles that occurs during walking and subsides with rest. It results from inadequate blood supply, which may be due to atherosclerosis or arterial spasm. Arterial cleansing relieves and eliminates all forms of leg pain that are caused by narrowing arteries.

Cholesterol may normalize. There is no direct relationship between elevated serum cholesterol and cardiovascular disease. Most people who have had heart attacks or strokes also had normal cholesterol levels at the time. Most people who have bypass surgery have normal cholesterol levels. The usual pattern is for plaque to build up on artery walls without any corresponding change in cholesterol levels in the blood itself.

The most effective ways to bring down high cholesterol involve drinking more water, increasing dietary fiber, eliminating sugar, getting more exercise, and normalizing thyroid function. Quite a number of people, however, have reported reductions in cholesterol readings as a side benefit of simply taking the arterial cleansing formula (ACF). When this happens, it may because nutrients in the ACF helped to correct whatever metabolic imbalance that was causing the elevated cholesterol (hypercholesterolemia). One writer explained it this way, "My cholesterol went down because my body no longer needs cholesterol to moderate the arterial damage".

Blood pressure may normalize. The vast majority of cases of high blood pressure (hypertension) are caused or aggravated by hidden food allergies. Almost any food or beverage can cause this response, depending on each person's unique sensitivities. The most frequent offenders in this regard, however, are caffeine and the nightshade family (tomatoes, potatoes, peppers, paprika, eggplant, cayenne, and tobacco). Blood pressure usually returns to normal within four days of eliminating 100 percent of the causative allergens.

Sometimes hypertension is caused by narrowing arteries that are losing elasticity. The heart has to pump harder in order to assure that the blood flows everywhere it can, causing blood pressure to increase. In such cases, arterial cleansing tends to restore blood pressure to normal.

Heart health maintained. The heart muscle (myocardium) receives its oxygen and nutrients through three arteries (right coronary artery, left coronary artery, circumflex artery). Blockages that accumulate in any of these small arteries eventually cause angina and heart attacks. Reducing such blockages before any adverse symptoms are experienced is prevention rather than therapy – prevention that ensures the heart continues to receive its critical supply of oxygen.

Reducing blockages throughout the arterial tree may ease the load on the heart: this muscular organ does not have to work quite so hard if it is no longer pushing against obstructions. There have also been a few cases in which it appears that the chelating ingredients in the ACF may have reduced calcification on heart valves. Heart murmurs have multiple possible causes unrelated to atherosclerosis and so do not respond to arterial cleansing.

General health improves. Arterial cleansing empowers the body to reduce and eliminate arterial plaque wherever it may occur. The circulatory system becomes more efficient, improving the blood's ability to bring oxygen and nutrients to bodily cells everywhere. The entire body benefits from improved circulation. Having more energy, looking younger, and sleeping better are the usual benefits experienced after the first three weeks on the program. Later benefits sometimes include improved vision, better prostate function, or increased libido.

A SCIENTIFIC EXPLANATION

Science is the intellectual process using all available mental and physical resources to better understand, explain and predict normal as well as unusual natural phenomena. The scientific approach to understanding anything involves observation, measurement of that which can be quantified, and the accumulation of data. [*Taber's Cyclopedic Medical Dictionary*]

Empirical science is based on observation and verifiable experience rather than theory or pure logic. The law of gravity was discovered and is completely verifiable by observation and experience, as is the fact that the earth revolves around the sun, and also the fact that citrus juices cure scurvy.

Epidemiology is that branch of science concerned with the incidence and distribution of health related states and events in populations. Epidemiology tells us that atherosclerosis has reached epidemic proportions and kills more people than all other disease causes combined.

From the above perspectives, the arterial cleansing formula (ACF) is on a solid scientific footing. Many thousands of people on three continents have been using this formula for over 30 years to remove arterial blockages, as evidenced by amelioration of their symptoms (e.g., no more angina, bypass surgery avoided, intermittent claudication gone, no more tingling sensations, warmer hands and feet, gangrene reversed) as well as by confirming ultrasound tests of coronary and carotid arteries. This is both empirical and epidemiological evidence of outstanding significance.

Repeatability and predictability are why science exists. When event A happens, we want to know what the outcome will be. The ACF meets all scientific standards of predictability. We know what happens when people take it. *The ACF is to atherosclerosis what oranges are to scurvy.*

EXPERIENTIAL PROOF

Experience is the ultimate proof. Everything else is only theory (a fancy word for supposition). We know that the arterial cleansing formula works because so many thousands of people have experienced its benefits. Because of biochemical individuality, responses to this formula vary from person to person. Those who are in reasonably good health may experience only subtle benefits, while others can overcome significant health conditions, thereby extending their lives and improving their quality of life. There have been only about 25 individuals over the last 30 years that have reported no perceptible benefits from taking the ACF. The only way to know if it will work for you is to try it. The answer to the question, "What proof do you have that the ACF works?" is "Take it and you will be the proof."

Theories come and go. At various times in history scientists believed that the world was flat, that the sun revolved around the earth, that bloodletting was a cure-all for whatever ails you, and that cholesterol causes heart disease. All four of these theories are false. The truth of an idea has nothing to do with its popularity. Sometimes the majority can be wrong.

Once a notion becomes entrenched, it can be difficult to see other possibilities. The tendency is to see only what you wish. Scientists refused to look through the lens of Galileo's foolish telescope because they were absolutely certain that the sun revolved around the earth. French doctors in the time of Jacques Cartier refused to believe that his men had been cured from scurvy by consuming pine needle tea. They said, "No. That can't work. That's witchcraft."

FIRST EVIDENCE OF DAMAGE

The first visual evidence we have of developing atherosclerosis is *what mistakenly appear to be* fatty streaks in the inner lining of arteries. Closer examination reveals that these streaks are <u>not</u> fats but rather dead macrophages (immune cells). These macrophages have become trapped in rough scar tissue caused by the healing of tiny cuts or tears in the arterial lining. Thus, the true cause of atherosclerosis is whatever damages the arterial wall. The most likely culprits are free radicals, homocysteine, and diabetes.

OXIDIZED CHOLESTEROL

A number of scientists who became disenchanted with the cholesterol theory decided to modify it somewhat. They observed that not all cholesterol in arterial deposits is the same; some of it has become oxidized. They speculated that it must be the oxidized cholesterol that causes the damage; and from this assumption followed a number of dietary precautions, such as cooking eggs over low heat so as not to damage their cholesterol content.

The oxidized cholesterol theory has two flaws: (1) oxidized cholesterol is one of the last ingredients laid down in the arterial plaque, not the first, and (2) it is more likely that this cholesterol became oxidized after it accumulated in the plaque. An outer layer of cholesterol may have sacrificed itself in order to protect deeper layers and the artery itself from further damage from oxygen free radicals. From this perspective, cholesterol could be considered an antioxidant of last resort.

179

INFLAMMATION

Inflammation is a nonspecific immune response that occurs in reaction to any type of bodily injury [*Taber's Cyclopedic Medical Dictionary*]. C-reactive protein (CRP) is a protein found in the blood, the levels of which rise in response to inflammation and are associated with atherosclerosis, diabetes, autoimmune disorders, and sports injuries. In other words, atherosclerosis raises CRP levels, but not all elevated CRP levels are triggered by atherosclerosis.

Arterial inflammation usually increases CRP levels before any significant blockages show up on ultra sound tests. This does not mean that inflammation causes atherosclerosis, however. Jumping to this kind of erroneous conclusion is known in logic as the *post hoc proper hoc* fallacy – meaning that just because one event precedes another does not prove that the former caused the latter. In scientific terms, this is the error of assuming that correlation is cause.

Inflammation is a symptom, not a cause. Inflammation does not cause atherosclerosis any more than inflammation causes arthritis or sports injuries. In all cases, inflammation is a response to damage of some kind. We need to find out what is causing the damage. With respect to atherosclerosis, the most likely causative agents are free radicals, homocysteine and elevated blood glucose (as in diabetes).

HYPOASCORBEMIA

We humans suffer from a genetic defect whereby our livers are incapable of producing ascorbate (vitamin C) the way that most mammals and birds do. Hypoascorbemia (insufficent vitamin C) is the reason why supplementary vitamin C is beneficial to so many health conditions. Here is a remarkable fact: animals which produce ascorbate in their livers do not develop atherosclerosis. If you wish to induce atherosclerosis in animals for research purposes, you have to use animals that also suffer from hypoascorbemia (e.g., monkeys or guinea pigs).

Somehow, the ability to produce vitamin C internally prevents an animal's arteries from plugging up. This is probably for at least three reasons: (1) vitamin C is required for the production of lipoprotein lipase (LPL), an arterial cleansing enzyme, (2) vitamin C is required for the production of Co-enzyme Q_{10}, an antioxidant that protects arteries from damaging oxygen free radicals, and (3) vitamin C is itself a powerful antioxidant. The implication is that by taking suitably high amounts of vitamin C throughout our entire lives, we may be able to prevent atherosclerosis. It is unlikely, however, that vitamin C supplementation alone would be capable of removing arterial plaque that has been accumulating over years.

LIPOPROTEIN LIPASE

Cholesterol, triglycerides, and phospholipids are lipoproteins, the molecules of which consist of fats chemically linked to proteins. Lipoproteins are classified as very low-density (VLDL), low-density (LDL), intermediate density (IDL), and high density (HDL). It is thought that individuals with high blood levels of HDL are less predisposed to coronary heart disease than those with high blood levels of VLDL or LDL. This is because the lower density lipoproteins are puffier and may readily block openings in tiny capillaries or in occluded arteries. The body's natural way of reducing excess lipoproteins is to make lipoprotein lipase.

Lipoprotein lipase (LPL) is a water soluble, fat splitting enzyme (i.e., an emulsifier) that hydrolyzes triglycerides in low density lipoproteins into free fatty acids and one monoacylglycerol molecule. It is also involved in promoting the cellular uptake of chylomicron remnants, cholesterol-rich lipoproteins, and free fatty acids. LPL is attached to the surface of some cells that line the capillaries and arteries, and is also distributed in adipose, heart and skeletal muscle tissue, as well as in lactating mammary glands.

Lipoprotein lipase works like a detergent to emulsify cholesterol and triglycerides, enabling them to be carried safely away through the liver and bile. There is a catch, however. Without adequate vitamin C, the human body cannot produce enough LPL to prevent excess fats and cholesterol from accumulating in arterial plaque.

LIPOPROTEIN(A)

Lipoprotein(a) is structurally similar to low density lipoproteins (LDL) and is often considered to be a marker for atherosclerotic diseases. In other words, if there is a significant lipoprotein(a) reading in your blood work, you are theoretically considered to be at higher risk of developing atherosclerosis than if your other lipoprotein fractions are out of balance. But there is a missing link in this chain of reasoning. Lipoprotein(a) may well indicate a genetic predisposition for elevated or distorted cholesterol readings. However, there is no conclusive scientific evidence that cholesterol or other lipoproteins actually cause atherosclerosis, plus a number of logical reasons why they cannot. [*See the chapter entitled "The Cholesterol Myth".*]

CO-ENZYME Q$_{10}$

Co-enzyme Q$_{10}$ (ubiquinone, ubiquinol) is a vitamin-like substance that is present in all bodily cells and generates energy in the form of adenosine triphosphate (ATP). CoQ$_{10}$ is abundant in organs with high energy requirements, such as the heart, liver and kidneys. CoQ$_{10}$ also functions as an antioxidant to protect cells against the damaging effects of oxygen free radicals. These combined actions of CoQ$_{10}$ help both to strengthen the heart muscle and also to prevent damage to arterial walls.

If the body has a sufficiently high intake of vitamin C and B-vitamins, it is capable of producing all of the CoQ$_{10}$ it needs – without resorting to dietary CoQ$_{10}$. Large amounts of vitamin C can also supplement and even replace the antioxidant activity of CoQ$_{10}$. Cholesterol lowering drugs interfere with and deplete the body's production of CoQ$_{10}$, however, so anyone taking these pharmaceuticals is well advised also to take supplementary CoQ$_{10}$.

FREE RADICALS

A free radical is an unstable, highly reactive molecular fragment that contains an odd number of electrons and an open bond or half bond. If two free radicals meet, both are eliminated. If a radical reacts with a nonradical, another free radical is produced. This type of event may become a chain reaction and may contribute to the development of ischemic injury, such as myocardial infarction (heart attack). Cascading free radical reactions appear to be the most significant cause of arterial damage.

NUTRITIONAL SOLUTIONS FOR 88 CONDITIONS

HOMOCYSTEINE

Homocysteine is a toxic amino acid that inflames and damages artery walls. Homocysteine is an intermediate by-product resulting from the incomplete breakdown (catabolism) of methionine, an amino acid that is abundant in our diet.

A high level of homocysteine in the blood (hyperhomocysteinemia) is associated with an increased risk of developing coronary artery disease, and may account for 60 percent of peripheral vascular diseases (i.e., those affecting the extremities). Men with hyperhomocysteinemia may have three times more heart attacks than those with low levels of homocysteine.

The ideal level of homocysteine in the blood is zero, and it is very easy to achieve this level. All that is necessary is to take sufficient levels of **vitamin B$_6$**, **vitamin B$_{12}$**, and **folic acid** – all of which vitamins are generously supplied in the ACF (arterial cleansing formula).

BLOOD SUGAR

All of the various sugars we consume are first broken down in the digestive tract into the simple sugars glucose (dextrose) and fructose (levulose), then immediately absorbed through the intestinal wall directly into the bloodstream. The liver converts fructose into glucose, so ultimately every kind of sugar ends up as glucose (blood sugar). If we consume too much sugar, our blood becomes flooded with excess levels of glucose. If our pancreas, liver and adrenal glands are in fine working order, then this spike in blood sugar is only temporary. If our endocrine system is out of balance and we push our sugar consumption, then we may develop hypoglycemia or diabetes. (Some forms of diabetes are caused or aggravated by genetic weakness.)

Hypoglycemia is characterized by compulsive sugar consumption which triggers multiple highs and lows in blood sugar throughout the day. In diabetes, blood sugar is constantly too high. Unfortunately, high glucose levels accelerate free radical damage – the degree of which damage is most probably in direct proportion to how high the glucose level and for how much of the day. In the development of arterial damage (a) diabetes is a hugely accelerating factor, (b) hypoglycemia is probably an aggravating factor, and (c) in otherwise healthy people, high sugar meals may cause some degree of arterial stress. Our bodies can get all of the glucose we need for optimal functioning from the gradual breakdown of complex carbohydrates (e.g., whole grains, starchy vegetables), thus avoiding spikes in blood sugar.

BLOOD FATS

The body has a very clever way of assuring that fats in the bloodstream stay within an acceptable range. The fats that we consume are broken down by the action of bile and lipase enzymes into simpler fatty acids that are absorbed into the lymphatic system rather than the bloodstream. To absorb fats directly into the blood would be fatal. Instead, fats circulate throughout the lymphatics and are transferred into the blood as needed, in a precisely regulated way. Thus, the quantity of dietary fats consumed is irrelevant to atherosclerosis. The quality of fats consumed, however, is an entirely different matter. Unstable polyunsaturated oils, rancid fats and *trans* fats circulating in our lymphatic system find their way into cellular membranes, thus increasing their vulnerability to free radical damage.

COMPOSITION OF ARTERIAL PLAQUE

Atheroma is an accumulation and swelling in artery walls made up of macrophage cells, debris, lipids (cholesterol and fatty acids), calcium and a variable amount of fibrous connective tissue. These accumulations are commonly referred to as atheromatous plaques. It is an unhealthy condition, but is found in most humans. Veins never develop atheroma, unless surgically moved to function as an artery, as in bypass surgery.

The atheromatous swelling is between the endothelium lining and the smooth muscle wall central region of the arterial tube. The early stages have been misdiagnosed as fatty streaks by pathologists; however, there is no fat in them. They are instead accumulations of white blood cells, especially macrophages. After accumulating large amounts of cytoplasmic membranes, these dead macrophages are called "foam cells". When foam cells die, their contents are released, which attracts more macrophages and creates an extracellular lipid core near the center to inner surface of each atherosclerotic plaque. The outer, older portions of the plaque become calcified.

The thickening of the walls of the arteries appears as an accumulation of soft, flaky, yellowish material with deposits of swollen macrophages as its bottom layer and a somewhat firmer coating on top. Interspersed in this accumulation can be seen fibrous tissue, calcium, cholesterol crystals, and fatty material. Some plaques are unstable and can rupture. Because of its spontaneous abnormal growth and swelling, the plaque loosely fits the definition of a benign tumor.

Macrophages are phagocytic immune cells that serve as the major scavengers in the blood, clearing it of diseased cells, cellular debris and pathogenic organisms. The question is why do macrophages make up such a large part of the atherosclerotic plaque? Why also are these white blood cells the first constituent of plaque to adhere to the artery wall? The clearest answer to both questions is that the macrophages are needed to dispose of arterial cells that have become damaged. Macrophages absorb damaged proteins and LDL cholesterol, then swell up to become foam cells that stick to the injured artery wall. The **vitamin A** and **thymus** concentrate in the ACF enable the thymus gland to increase production of macrophages, thus facilitating the cleanup of damaged arterial cells.

What is this fibrous connective tissue that is also a significant component of arterial plaque? Most probably it is the result of blood platelets doing their job. When a blood vessel is injured, platelets adhere to each other and the edges of the injury and form a plug that covers the area. This leads to enhancement of the coagulation mechanism and deposition of fibrin. The plug that is formed acts like a scab that retracts to stop the loss of blood The actions of platelets, although quite beneficial in initiating the reaction to injury, may actually be harmful in conditions such as coronary occlusion. In that case, platelet function may delay restoration of the blood supply and help to cause re-occlusion of the vessel. Healthy platelets are critical to the healing of the artery wall; but unhealthy platelets tend to stick to each other excessively, thus adding unnecessary bulk to the arterial plaque. **Vitamin E** keeps platelets healthy and prevents them from unduly sticking together.

Fibrin is a whitish, filamentous protein that is the basis for blood clotting. This fibrin is deposited as fine interlacing filaments, containing entangled red and white blood cells and platelets, the whole forming a coagulum or clot. In other words, fibrin acts like a scab to prevent a cut or tear from bleeding out or hemorrhaging – and also traps calcium ions before they can form lumps of calcium that would plug arteries and capillaries. This rough scab-like structure on the artery wall becomes a matrix in which are trapped minerals, heavy metals, macrophages, cellular debris, fats, and cholesterol from the bloodstream – substances that could not possibly adhere to the smooth lining of a healthy artery.

Minerals and fats attract each other, because of opposing electromagnetic charges. Minerals from the bloodstream become trapped in arterial scar tissue and attract fats electromagnetically. These fats become an integral part of the accumulating plaque, and in turn attract more minerals, especially calcium – and so on, repeating the cycle and ever increasing the size of the plaque.

CELLULAR INTEGRITY

Atherosclerosis occurs only in arteries, never in veins. This is because of the structural differences between artery cells and vein cells.

Every cell in our bodies is enclosed in a membrane that separates the interior of cells from their outside environment. This cellular membrane selectively controls what molecules may enter and exit the cell. The basic function of the cellular membrane is to protect the cell from its surroundings.

Most cellular membranes consist of about 50 percent lipids (fats), depending on the type of cell. These lipids are in two layers which behave as fluids in which individual molecules (both lipids and proteins) are free to rotate and move. Such fluidity of membranes is greatly affected by lipid composition. Lipids containing unsaturated fatty acids increase membrane fluidity because the presence of loose double carbon bonds introduces kinks in the fatty acid chains, making them more difficult to pack together. Cholesterol in membranes also increases fluidity. What all this means is that the more unsaturated fatty acids and cholesterol a cellular membrane contains, the more fluid or flexible it is.

Because monounsaturated fatty acids (i.e., omega-9) have only one double carbon bond in their structure, they are more stable and less fluid than unsaturated fatty acids. Thus, omega-9 fatty acids contribute stability to cellular membranes. Oleic acid is the primary omega-9 fatty acid in our cellular membranes and is provided in large amounts by olive oil, almond oil, macadamia oil, avocado oil and cashew oil.

Arteries are the high pressure tubes of the circulatory system. They contain an extra muscular layer that the veins do not. These arterial muscles are constantly flexing, pushing blood along. In order to maintain this flexibility, artery cells have to be more fluid than most other cells in the body – meaning that they necessarily have to contain a relatively high percentage of unsaturated fats – and therein lies their vulnerability. Unsaturated fats are unstable and highly susceptible to free radical damage because of the large number of weak double carbon bonds in their molecular structure.

In order to maintain needed flexibility, artery cells contain a high proportion of unstable unsaturated fats and a low percentage of the stable, protective monounsaturates. The body does its best to maintain a favorable ratio of unsaturates to monounsaturates in arterial cells; however, its ability to do so is limited by diet. If we do not consume enough monounsaturates, then the body has no choice but to fill cellular membranes with even more unsaturates than is healthy or desirable, thus making the arteries structurally weaker and more vulnerable to free radical damage than they would otherwise be. The more polyunsaturated oils we consume, the more vulnerable our arteries tend to become.

It is ironic that the highly promoted polyunsaturated oils (e.g., safflower, sunflower, corn, soy, walnut, flax, pumpkin) may actually contribute to the development of atherosclerosis if consumed to excess. Consistent with this theory is epidemiological evidence which shows that in Mediterranean countries where olive oil (79 percent monounsaturate) is a staple, the incidence of heart disease is significantly lower than it is elsewhere.

If a blood clot suddenly plugs up a narrowed coronary artery, this immediate deprivation of blood usually causes an instant heart attack. If the blood supply to the heart's internal pacemaker is suddenly cut off, then that heart attack is fatal. If other areas of the heart are suddenly deprived of blood, and provided the damage is not too extensive, the result is usually a non-fatal heart attack.

If a coronary artery narrows gradually and provided there is enough **vitamin E** present, the body is often able to develop collateral circulation. This phenomenon was discovered during autopsies and cardiac surgeries which revealed previously unknown arterial blockages for which the body had apparently created its own bypasses.

This is the body's innate wisdom at its finest. As a coronary artery slowly narrows, small arteries (arterioles) gradually extend into the area that is about to be deprived of its usual blood source – with incredible timing. By the time the affected artery becomes 100 percent blocked, the backup system is already in place; and the heart remains as healthy as ever.

A client once came to me with laboratory confirmed collateral bypasses. Multiple tests showed that one of his coronary arteries was 100 percent blocked and that his heart had also developed collateral circulation that negated the problem. Although this man was not especially fit, he managed to pass two treadmill stress tests with flying colors – no shortness of breath, no ECG abnormalities. His cardiologist told him that his heart was in great shape; and there was no need to be concerned about the blocked artery, which to the doctor seemed to be nothing more than an interesting anomaly.

ARTERIAL SPASMS

Apart from accumulating plaque, arteries can fail in an entirely different way. Spasms in healthy coronary arteries can temporarily restrict blood supply to the heart, causing angina, a heart attack, and/or death. In death, the artery relaxes so that an autopsy will be unable to find any apparent cause for the heart attack. **Magnesium** prevents arterial spasms.

A client complained to me about repeated angina that she had learned to control by eating chocolate, a rich source of magnesium. There were no indications of any actual arterial blockages anywhere in her body. Whenever she experienced angina, she ate some chocolate and it always went away. After learning this relationship, she switched from chocolate bars to magnesium tablets, with always the same beneficial results.

A PLAUSIBLE THEORY

From the above scientific observations, we can piece together a theory that (a) is more plausible than any others advanced to date, and (b) is consistent with many thousands of successful experiences with arterial cleansing. There are three parts to this theory: (1) atherosclerosis is caused by agents that damage artery walls, (2) the body does what it can to control the damage, the unfortunate consequence of which is the accumulation of plaque that gradually occludes arteries, and (3) certain high potency nutrients enable the body both to prevent arterial occlusion and also to reverse that which has already taken place. Key elements in this theory:

- Free radicals and homocysteine create tiny tears in the inner lining of artery walls.
- Excess blood sugar accelerates this arterial damage.
- The body patches arterial tears with fibrin (a clotting protein) and scarring.
- Dead macrophages (immune cells) become trapped in the patches and scar tissue.
- These macrophages swell up to become foam cells
- Through time, more and more substances become attracted to and trapped in the arterial patches – including collagen, fats, minerals (especially calcium), foreign proteins, heavy metals, phospholipids, mucopolysaccharides, muscle tissue, cellular debris, triglycerides, and cholesterol.
- The parts of the arterial tree most vulnerable to the accumulation of plaque are the coronary arteries, the carotid arteries, and the femoral arteries.
- Plaque that is allowed to proliferate out of control eventually causes a heart attack, a stroke, or gangrene.
- Antioxidants protect the arteries from the damaging effects of oxygen free radicals. (An antioxidant is a molecule that can absorb a renegade electron without becoming a free radical itself.) Dietary antioxidants include **vitamin C**, **vitamin E**, and **selenium**.
- **Vitamin C** and the **B-vitamins** encourage the body to make coenzyme Q_{10}, an internally generated antioxidant.
- **Selenium**, **zinc** and **manganese** facilitate the body's production of free radical scavengers.
- **Vitamins B_6, B_{12}** and **folic acid** eliminate the homocysteine hazard.
- **Vitamin C** in large amounts encourages the arteries to produce LPL, an enzyme that emulsifies and disposes of fats that have accumulated in artery walls.
- Certain high potency nutrients act as chelating agents to remove minerals and heavy metals from arterial plaque – including **vitamin C**, **L-cysteine**, **DL-methionine**, and **thiamine**.
- **Magnesium** dissolves calcium deposits in arterial plaque.
- **Magnesium** also prevents arterial spasms, some of which can be fatal.
- Large amounts of **vitamin E** encourage the body to develop collateral circulation, in effect creating self-generated bypasses.

- **Choline** emulsifies fats, keeping them from sticking together and thereby improving the flow characteristics of the blood.
- **Vitamin E** prevents blood platelets from sticking together, thus reducing their tendency to contribute to excessive coagulation in arterial patches.
- **Monounsaturated oils** (e.g., olive, avocado, almond) have a protective effect on arterial cell membranes.

FATS AND OILS

Contrary to popular myth, saturated fats do ***not*** cause heart disease. If they did, the rural populations of western countries would have died off generations ago due to their high consumption of beef, pork, bacon, eggs, sausages, lard, etc. Natural fats that are predominately saturated are extremely stable and can still provide tiny amounts of essential fatty acids.

Similarly, polyunsaturated oils do ***not*** prevent heart disease. They probably contribute to it. Polyunsaturated oils are chemically unstable. This is because they have multiple loose double carbon bonds in their molecular structure. When subject to heat or air, they oxidize rapidly to form harmful free radicals. The more unsaturated the oil, the more potentially hazardous it is. Oils that are predominately unsaturated include hemp, safflower, sunflower, corn, soy, wheat germ, walnut, flax, pumpkin and cottonseed.

The most hazardous vegetable oils are those used by restaurants for deep frying. These oils are heated and re-heated many times over. They are rancid; however, you cannot smell the rancidity because of deodorants added by the manufacturers.

Other hazardous oils are those which have been hydrogenated to form margarine, shortening or other commercially modified fats. They contain peroxidized fats, *trans* fatty acids, and other artificial fat molecules which can compromise immune processes in the body.

Even the so called "cold pressed" oils can be harmful, due to the heat (over 100°C) generated by the friction of the processing equipment. As soon as they are exposed to air these oils degenerate rapidly; and when used for cooking, their destruction is assured.

Healthy fatty acids are crucial to our well-being. They help to form the membranes that surround every cell in the body. (Healthy cell membranes are part of our immune defenses against degenerative diseases.) Fatty acids are precursors to hormone-like substances called "prostaglandins", which help to regulate gastric secretions, pancreatic functions, and the release of pituitary hormones. Fatty acids combine with glycerol to form triglycerides, which act as carriers for vitamins A, D and E and help to convert beta carotene into vitamin A.

Fatty acids are of three basic types: <u>saturated</u> (e.g., palmitic acid, stearic acid), <u>monounsaturated</u> (e.g., oleic acid), and <u>polyunsaturated</u> (e.g., linoleic, linolenic, arachidonic). All of the fats and oils we consume consist of various proportions of these three groups. For example, ghee (clarified butter) is approximately 68 percent saturated, 27 percent monounsaturated, and five percent polyunsaturated. Olive oil is approximately 13 percent saturated, 79 percent monounsaturated, and eight percent polyunsaturated.

If our diets provide an adequate supply of all of the basic fatty acids, our bodies can select the best ones for the tasks that need to be accomplished on any given day. If the best ones are not available, then our bodies are compelled to do the best they can with whatever is available. This is how the integrity of cellular membranes becomes compromised. Arterial cell walls require a certain percentage of oleic acid (monounsaturated) in their membranes in order to resist deterioration from free radicals. If, however, we have not consumed sufficient monounsaturates and our bodies also have not been able to de-saturate enough saturated fats to make sufficient oleic acid, then our arterial cell membranes contain too high a percentage of the unstable polyunsaturates thus increasing their susceptibility to free radical damage.

There are only two essential fatty acids: linoleic acid (omega-6) and alpha-linolenic acid (omega-3). If we have a sufficient intake of these two – and in the presence of sufficient vitamins and minerals – the body can make all of the other fatty acids it needs. [*"Essential" means "indispensable" and applies only to nutrients they must be supplied from food because our bodies cannot manufacture them.*]

The essential fatty acids we require are found in relatively high proportions in polyunsaturated oils. This creates for us a balancing act, because the polyunsaturates are the ones most prone to deterioration from free radicals. Fortunately, those fats and oils that are predominantly saturated or monounsaturated also contain smaller but significant amounts of essential fatty acids.

Because it is not an essential fatty acid, the very important role of oleic acid (omega-9) in stabilizing cellular membranes has been largely overlooked. There is a tenuous assumption that the body should be able to make all of the omega-9 it needs if its intake of omega-3 and omega-6 fats is adequate. This happens only if conditions are ideal, and they rarely are. Mediterranean countries tend to use olive oil as a dietary staple. Doing so ensures that the body has an adequate intake of oleic acid without having to convert other fatty acids. Thus, omega-9 spares the action of omega-3's and omega-6's, leaving them available for other purposes. The incidence of heart disease is significantly lower in countries where consumption of olive oil is relatively high. Not a coincidence.

Oleic acid (omega-9) is a monounsaturated fatty acid. This means that it has only one loose double carbon bond in its molecular structure, making it much more resistant to deterioration than the polyunsaturates. Oils that are high in mononunsaturates include olive, macadamia, avocado, cashew, hickory, hazelnut/filbert, pecan, and pistachio.

Fish body oils are a source of intermediate omega-3 fatty acids, the principal one of which is EPA (eicosapentaenoic acid). EPA improves the flow characteristics of blood by preventing blood cells from sticking together to form clots that might otherwise prematurely plug narrowed arteries. EPA also tends (a) to reduce serum cholesterol levels, and (b) to increase HDL cholesterol (the "good" kind). EPA is nature's anti-freeze, to keep the fish's body from stiffening in cold temperatures. The colder the water the fish lives in, the higher its EPA content. Most fish will do, with some of the best sources being salmon, mackerel, krill, cod, herring, haddock, trout, whitefish, oysters, and squid.

Organic flax oil is used therapeutically to treat a number of conditions. It provides approximately 57 percent alpha-linolenic acid (omega-3), 16 percent linoleic acid (omega-6), and 18 percent oleic acid (omega-9). Raw flaxseed oil, however, is highly susceptible to deterioration because of its 73 percent content of polyunsaturates. A healthier choice is flaxseed oil that has been specially processed at 40^0 C in a controlled atmosphere of nitrogen (rather than oxygen), hermetically sealed into opaque capsules, and packaged in light-resistant bottles – all of this to resist the destructive influences of oxygen and light.

Both the quantity and quality of fats and oils we consume are critical to health. If our total fat intake is too low, we do not have enough essential fatty acids to thrive and we increase our risk for degenerative diseases. If our total fat intake is too high, the body uses first the fatty acids it can most readily assimilate, leaving the less desirable and unstable ones to circulate throughout the lymphatic system, contributing to tissue damage in various locations.

There are many dietary supplements that have positive benefits for the cardiovascular system, including: vitamin E, omega-3 oils, L-carnitine, magnesium, coenzyme Q_{10}, garlic, and hawthorne. All of these are beneficial in ameliorating symptoms of cardiovascular diseases. None of these, however, whether taken singly or in combination with any of the others is capable of correcting the cause of arterial blockages. The only dietary supplement capable of reducing atherosclerotic buildup is a high potency combination of select vitamins, minerals, amino acids, and glandular concentrates generically known as the arterial cleansing formula (ACF). Many people attribute the ACF with having saved or extended their lives.

NUTRITIONAL BYPASS PROGRAM

What you are about to read has transformed many lives and saved countless others. It is a program that provides your body with the raw materials and conditions to re-engage its innate healing abilities. In the 1980s it was called the "arterial cleansing" program. In the 1990s it became known as "the nutritional bypass". The complete nutritional bypass program involves three key elements:

1. Reducing exposure to harmful factors,
2. Increasing intake of foods that have a protective effect, and
3. A broad spectrum of specific high potency supplements.

It is important that physical exercise also be included in any nutritional bypass program. Regular exercise is both protective of our cardiovascular system and supportive of immune processes. It tones muscles, eases stress, stimulates internal organs, relieves depression, helps to lower cholesterol, improves lymphatic flow, and helps one to think more clearly. The best form of exercise is one which you enjoy and will cause you to sweat for at least 30 minutes, repeated three times per week. Rapid walking, cycling, aerobics, racquet sports, team sports, martial arts – anything that can raise your pulse rate to between 120 and 140 beats per minute. Exercise tones the cardiovascular system but does not reduce arterial blockages, however.

There have been a number of world class athletes who have dropped dead from heart attacks.

Guidelines to follow when implementing the full program:

1. Stop smoking and/or avoid second hand tobacco smoke.
2. Reduce exposure to radiation, X-rays, exhaust fumes, and industrial pollutants.
3. Drink at least 8 glasses of purified water daily. Avoid drinking or bathing in chlorinated water.
4. Use olive oil and butter as primary fats/oils. Reduce intake of polyunsaturated oils. Avoid rancid fats/oils, deep fried foods, margarines, shortening, and *trans* fats.
5. Eat fish twice weekly and/or supplement with omega-3 fish body oils.
6. Restrict concentrated sugars of all kinds (sucrose, glucose, fructose, white sugar, brown sugar, raw sugar, corn syrup, maple syrup, honey, molasses, fruit juices, etc.).
7. Limit alcoholic beverages to two drinks per week.
8. Limit caffeine intake (coffee, tea, colas) to the equivalent of one cup of coffee or two cups of tea (preferably green tea) daily.
9. Avoid processed meats, nitrates, nitrites and other suspect food preservatives.
10. Take the arterial cleansing formula (ACF).

The first nine recommendations above provide a nutritional environment as close as possible to our pre-1910 ancestors, all of whom were apparently immune to heart attacks. Reducing risk factors addresses only one part of the problem, however. The other part requires strengthening immune processes not only to withstand future insults, but also to clear away the arterial plaque that has been accumulating over the years. This is the purpose of the tenth item on the above list.

ARTERIAL CLEANSING FORMULA

The human body has an incredible, innate ability to heal itself – provided we give it what it needs to do the job. We are subject to more cardiovascular risks than our heart-disease-free ancestors, and our bodies are less well equipped to deal with them. Our dependence on agribusiness and processed foods leaves us lacking in vital nutrients required for healthy immune function. Our stressful lifestyles significantly increase our bodies' needs for vital nutrients at a time when those nutrients are less available in our foods. Through time, our bodies have become both (a) exposed to more free radicals than ever before, and (b) less able to counteract those free radicals. The good news is that we can return our bodies to the natural cardio-protective state that our ancestors enjoyed. For over 30 years, many thousands of people have been doing just that – by taking the arterial cleansing formula (ACF) – a high potency, broad spectrum of nutrients that stimulate the body's innate processes both to clear away arterial plaque and to prevent its return. It works in the following ways:

1. Neutralizing free radicals before they can cause damage.
2. Protecting vital tissues from oxidative damage.
3. Eliminating homocysteine.
4. Making T-cells and macrophages to destroy mutated and damaged cells before they can accumulate in the arteries.
5. Making lipoprotein lipase (LPL) to emulsify and clear away fats from artery walls.
6. Chelating calcium, other minerals and heavy metals from artery walls.
7. Improving the flow characteristics (viscosity) of the blood.
8. Opening up collateral blood vessels around obstructions, creating new pathways for blood to reach vital tissues.
9. Dissolving blood clots.
10. Preventing arterial spasms.

Only a comprehensive, high potency formula in a very specific synergistic combination can accomplish all of the above. All other approaches to cardio-protective supplementation are fragmentary and exclude a number of vital links in the nutritional chain.

NUTRIENTS REQUIRED

The following is list of 19 key players on the arterial cleansing team. There are 8 other nutrients required in a supportive role, to enable the body to make the most efficient use of these 19. For best results, all 27 need to be present in optimal amounts.

Vitamin A. Stimulates the thymus gland to grow in size and enables it to produce more T-cells and antibodies. Increase utilization of selenium, an antioxidant.

Vitamin B-1. Facilitates removal of lead from tissues. Required for health of heart tissue.

Niacin. Helps the body to eliminate excess cholesterol.

Pantothenic Acid. Necessary for the production of healthy antibodies.

Vitamin B-6. Helps prevent methionine (a dietary amino acid) from breaking down into homocysteine, a toxic substance that can damage artery walls.

Vitamin B-12. Assists vitamin B-6 in eliminating homocysteine.

Folic Acid. Assists vitamins B-6 and B-12 in eliminating homocysteine.

Choline. Emulsifies fats that are released from the artery walls, keeping them in solution, preventing them from plugging up in narrowed arteries. Keeps fats in the blood from sticking together. Oxidizes or burns fats in the liver.

Vitamin C. A powerful antioxidant and chelating agent. Protects against heavy metals (e.g., lead, arsenic) and keeps them in solution so that they can be eliminated via the urine. Stimulates the production of lipoprotein lipase (LPL), an enzyme that dissolves fats on artery walls. Facilitates the body's internal production of coenzyme Q_{10}.

Vitamin E. A fat-soluble antioxidant. Protects against free radicals – including superoxides, hydroxyl radicals, peroxides, and hydroperoxides. Helps prevent and also dissolves clots in the blood. Improves the body's ability to grow collateral blood vessels around damaged areas. Helps keep blood platelets from sticking together.

Manganese. A free radical inhibitor.

Magnesium. Keeps calcium in solution, preventing it from being deposited in arterial plaque. Dissolves calcium in arterial plaque. Helps to regulate heartbeat. Prevents arterial spasms.

Potassium. Helps to normalize blood pressure. Helps to regulate heartbeat.

Zinc. A free radical inhibitor. Helps utilize vitamin A.

Selenium. 200 to 500 times more potent than vitamin E as an antioxidant. The body incorporates it into glutathione peroxidase, an antioxidant enzyme that detoxifies hydrogen peroxide and fatty acid peroxides. Assists vitamin E in inhibiting free radicals and protecting tissues from oxidative damage.

L-Cysteine Hydrochloride. An amino acid that acts as a chelating agent. Assists in the termination of free radicals produced by ionizing radiation.

DL-Methionine. A chelating agent and free radical scavenger. An amino acid that helps to detoxify the body and emulsify fats.

Thymus substance. Glandular tissue that supports thymus function, to produce T-cells that dispose of cells that have been damaged by free radicals.

POTENCIES REQUIRED

Thirty years of experience indicate that in order to achieve optimal arterial cleansing one needs to take all of the following supplemental nutrients daily, within the ranges recommended beside each. There is no one miracle ingredient in this formula. It is this very special combination of all 27, working together in synergistic orchestration that produces the results.

Needless to say, it is not possible to fit all of the above nutrients into a single tablet that is capable of being swallowed. It is necessary either (a) to piece together many tablets/capsules of fragmentary supplements, or (b) to take 10 tablets per day of a homogeneous supplement which combines all 27 nutrients in the proportions below.

Vitamin A	22,000 to 40,000 I.U.
Vitamin D	40 to 65 I.U.
Vitamin C	4,000 to 4,400 mg.
Vitamin E	600 to 650 I.U.
Vitamin B-1 (thiamine)	66 to 200 mg.
Vitamin B-2 (riboflavin)	30 to 55 mg.
Vitamin B-6 (pyridoxine)	50 to 150 mg.
Vitamin B-12`	160 to 550 mcg.
Niacin	44 to 70 mg.
Niacinamide	20 to 50 mg.
Pantothenic Acid	330 to 550 mg.
Folic Acid	0.4 to 2.2 mg.
Biotin	50 to 122 mg.
Choline (bitartrate)	440 to 725 mg.
Inositol	40 to 55 mg.
DL-Methionine	160 to 550 mg.
Magnesium (oxide)	400 to 555 mg.
Potassium (chloride)	400 to 444 mg.
Manganese (gluconate)	5 to 22 mg.
Zinc (gluconate)	25 to 33 mg.
Chromium (chelated)	130 to 333 mcg.
Selenium (chelated)	200 to 330 mcg.
Betaine hydrochloride	120 to 130 mg.
L-Cysteine hydrochloride	660 to 1,000 mg.
Thymus concentrate	55 to 100 mg.
Spleen concentrate	55 to 100 mg.
Adrenal concentrate	40 to 100 mg.

PROTOCOL

To achieve optimal arterial cleansing, it is usually necessary to take the equivalent of 10 of the homogeneous ACF tablets daily for one month for every 10 years of age (i.e., 4 months for someone aged 40, 6 months for someone aged 60, etc.) When this initial cleansing is completed, it is recommended to stay on a maintenance level of 5 tablets per day, in order to prevent the plaque from returning. Many people on this maintenance program like to bump up their intake to 10 tablets per day for a month or two every year, analogous to a spring cleaning.

Because diabetics are at such a high risk for arterial damage it is best for them to stay on the equivalent of 10 tablets of the ACF daily forever. Anyone who has had a heart attack, stroke or bypass surgery will have scarring left behind after the plaque has been removed. For this reason, they also are well advised to stay on 10 tablets per day for life. Scars tend to attract debris, thus re-initiating the buildup of arterial plaque.

The most efficient way to utilize the ACF is to take the 10 tablets per day in divided amounts with meals. This could be 3 tablets with breakfast, 4 with lunch, 3 with supper – or 5 with breakfast, 5 with supper. It is important to take the tablets with food so that the nutrients in the meal and the nutrients in the tablets support and enhance each other.

DIGESTIVE SUPPORT

Taking 10 tablets per day of the ACF should turn the urine a bright yellow color. This is caused by a tiny percentage of vitamin C that spills over into the urine. Pale urine while taking the ACF indicates digestive weakness – the tablets are not being broken down and absorbed from the digestive tract. The solution in this case is to take supplementary digestive enzymes with each meal. The most effective digestive support formula is one that includes betaine hydrochloride and bile plus a broad spectrum of protease, amylase and lipase enzymes. Take as many digestive aid tablets per meal as required to bring a bright yellow color to the urine.

FREQUENTLY ASKED QUESTIONS

Does the arterial cleansing formula work for everyone?

> Over the past 30 years there have been approximately 25 reports where the person taking the ACF received no perceptible benefits. In most of these cases there was an underlying digestive weakness indicated by pale colored urine (i.e., not breaking down the tablets and absorbing the nutrients). In other cases, the person's hyper-stressful

lifestyle may have overridden any benefit that the ACF might have been able to provide. One gentleman was constantly on the go, pushed himself to do one task after the other, ate on the run, never took time to rest; EDTA chelation therapy was not able to help him either.

How long will it take to feel any results on the arterial cleansing program?

This is a variable. We are all different. Most people start to notice slight improvements in about three weeks – such as having more energy, better skin tone, and requiring less sleep. Some are able to get complete relief from their angina or leg pains in about six weeks. Optimal arterial cleansing usually takes about one month for every 10 years of age, taking 10 ACF tablets consistently every day, and making sure that the urine turns bright yellow.

Are there any side effects to arterial cleansing?

Not as such. The ingredients in the formula are natural and safe. About five percent of people, however, may have temporary cleansing reactions lasting for up to 10 days – including headaches, nausea, indigestion, diarrhea, fatigue, or excessive intestinal gas. These signs indicate that the eliminative systems of the body are catching up with the release of debris from the plaque. During such cleansing reactions there are two choices: (1) reduce the number of tablets to 3 per day, then each day add one more tablet, gradually working back up to 10, or (2) continue on the 10 tablets per day knowing that the cleansing reaction will soon subside.

Will the arterial cleansing formula conflict with any prescription drugs I am taking?

There is no known conflict between the nutrients in the ACF and any prescription drugs, with the possible exception that some antibiotics tend to cancel out vitamin

C, and vice versa – in which case taking the antibiotics two hours apart from the ACF eliminates the conflict. If you are on prescribed medication, you need to have it monitored by your doctor. As your body gradually improves on the ACF, you will likely require less of your prescribed drugs. Your doctor and your pharmacist are the professionals qualified to counsel you about your drugs.

I am scheduled for bypass surgery in three weeks. Should I call off the surgery and try the arterial cleansing program instead?

This is a judgment call that only you can make. It is unlikely that the ACF can remove significant blockages in only three weeks. If the surgery can be postponed for at least three months, that would give the ACF a much better opportunity to prove its worth. If you opt for the surgery, then know that the ACF will help fortify your body to go through the operation, to heal faster, to prevent plaque from recurring where the blood vessels have been sutured, and also to remove plaque in areas not accessible to the surgeon.

Will the arterial cleansing formula pull away chunks of plaque that could plug up further downstream?

Absolutely not. The plaque is scrubbed away, safely and gradually, with a detergent-like action. There are enough emulsifiers (e.g., choline, methionine) in the ACF to keep fats in solution so that they do not plug up elsewhere.

Is it a good idea to take aspirin-like drugs during the arterial cleansing program? I have heard that ASA/aspirin helps to prevent heart attacks by making the blood thinner.

Most people do not have blood which is too thick, but rather blood cells which tend to clump or stick together. In addition to everything else the ACF does, it also improves the viscosity (slipperiness) of the blood, enabling it to flow more freely. Additional supplements of omega-3 fish body oils can sometimes further improve the blood's flow characteristics (viscosity).

CANCER IS A SYMPTOM

Question: What is the difference between a malignant cell and a healthy cell?

Answer: Not much. A cancerous cell is a normal cell that has become mutated.

Cancer is an imprecise term used to describe about 200 different kinds of neoplasms (tumors or abnormal growths) which serve no useful function but grow uncontrollably at the expense of healthy tissue. Carcinomas are cancers that grow in skin and in the linings and passageways of the body. Sarcomas grow in connective tissues, muscles, and skeleton. Leukemias are formed in bone marrow and affect the blood. "Malignant" is the term used to distinguish cancerous tumors from those which are benign or harmless.

Cancer is the second leading cause of death in North America. Its warning signs can include (1) change in bowel or bladder habits, (2) sores that do not heal, (3) unusual bleeding or discharge, (4) thickening or lump in breast or elsewhere, (5) indigestion or difficulty in swallowing, (6) obvious change in a wart or mole, or (7) nagging cough or hoarseness – all of which can also have other causes.

All of the various forms of cancer have the same cause: weakened immunity. Cancerous cells are created in every human body from time-to-time. If immune processes are strong, these malignant cells are quickly consumed by specialized white blood cells (phagocytes, leukocytes, macrophages) whose job it is to dispose of cellular debris. Cancer can take hold at a particular site only if one's immune system is weak. As immunity becomes progressively weaker, more malignant growths may appear in other parts of the body. The nutritional treatment of cancer thus requires giving the body the raw materials it needs to strengthen its immune processes.

According to Johns Hopkins University, every person may have cancer cells in the body on six or more occasions during a lifetime; but these mutated cells do not show up in standard tests until they have multiplied to a few billion. When the person's immune system is strong, the malignant cells are destroyed before they can form tumors.

Seen from this perspective, cancer is not a disease but a symptom. If you want relief from any symptom, then you have to correct the conditions which caused it. In the case of cancer, this means supporting and strengthening the body's innate immune processes.

BREAST CANCER

Breast cancer is the leading cause of death in women between the ages of 30 and 50, and is second only to heart disease as a cause of death in women over 50. The factor which appears to contribute the most to breast cancer is the brassiere. Women who never wear a bra have the same incidence of breast cancer as men. Women who wear a bra for 12 hours per day have over 20 times the rate of breast cancer as those who never wear a bra. Those who wear a bra for 24 hours a day have 100 times the rate of breast cancer as those who never wear a bra. The human breast is composed of large amounts of lymphatic tissue, which needs to drain continually in order to remain healthy. Lymph, however, cannot drain when it is compressed and restricted.

MEDICAL OPTIONS

Chemotherapy, radiation and surgery all attack the symptom. In cases where these modalities are successful at getting rid of tumors, cancer tends to recur. Why? Because these extreme measures do nothing to correct the true cause, weakened immunity.

Chemotherapy has the downside of itself weakening immunity. To give chemotherapy to a healthy person is to increase that person's risk of developing cancer. In cases where chemotherapy is successful at getting rid of tumors, it is often at the expense of increasing that person's susceptibility to new tumors popping up elsewhere.

A cancerous cell was once a healthy cell whose DNA became mutated, causing that cell to proliferate out of control. Malignant cells have the same content of proteins and essential fats as do healthy cells. Thus, chemotherapy poisons both cancerous cells and healthy cells.

According to Johns Hopkins University, chemotherapy poisons rapidly-growing cancer cells but also destroys rapidly-growing healthy cells in the bone marrow and gastrointestinal tract; and can also cause organ damage to liver, kidneys, heart, or lungs. Radiation kills malignant cells but also burns, scars and damages healthy cells, tissues and organs. Initial treatment with chemotherapy and radiation often reduce tumor size; however, prolonged use of these modalities does <u>not</u> result in further tumor destruction. In other words, past a certain point chemo and radiation only damage healthy cells without having any further effect on the cancer.

Some forms of cancer, such as basal cell carcinomas on the skin, respond well to surgery. As long as all of the papules and their margins are completely removed, there is never any recurrence at the same site (unless it is re-exposed to the same intensity of ultra violet radiation that caused the first carcinoma).

Heroic forms of surgery need to be considered very carefully. If a tumor is not life threatening, has stopped growing, is not applying pressure on a vital organ, is not impeding nerve or blood flow, then why have it removed at all? The tumor is merely a symptom. Rather than undergo a high risk operation to get rid of a symptom, it makes more sense to treat the cause by strengthening immunity. The great benefit of natural cancer therapies is that not only do they help to shrink tumors, they also prevent their recurrence – something that neither radiation, chemotherapy, nor surgery can do.

Cancer is a wakeup call that you have been either under-nourishing your immune system or overwhelming it, or both. Even if you are successful in having all of your tumors removed by radiation, chemo or surgery, that is not the end. It is just the beginning. Use the opportunity to find out how to empower your body's immune processes.

THE MYTH OF METASTASIS

Metastasis is a misconception. Because cancer first develops in one part of the body, then later may show up in other places, it is assumed that somehow malignant cells from the original tumor must have broken away, travelled through the blood or lymphatic system, and then planted roots in a new location. There are three things wrong with this speculative theory: (1) there is not one documented case where scientists have actually seen malignant cells in transit from one location to another, (2) cancerous cells are mutations generated from within the body; they are not bacteria-like invaders that attack whatever may be in their path, and (3) a tumor in a particular organ may grow incredibly large and put pressure on adjacent structures, but the tumor itself does not engulf adjacent tissues that are unrelated to the host organ. If malignant cells do not "infect" adjacent tissues, how can they be presumed to infect cells at remote locations?

Metastasis may describe some bacterial phenomena but has no relevance to cancer. When tumors gradually show up at different multiple sites, this is a symptom of a progressively weakening immune system. It is that simple.

EMOTIONAL CLIMATE

Dominant emotions affect our health. People who are really happy rarely get sick. Hard driving "type A" personalities increase their risk for cardiovascular diseases. There is also an emotional climate that increases one's susceptibility to cancer.

Those who develop cancer invariably do not feel entitled to express negative feelings. They may be outgoing, pleasant, affable – or indrawn and stoic – but you'll never know what is eating away at them emotionally. These people keep a lid on their negative feelings, letting them build up inside. "You can't fight city hall" and "He's such a nice guy, who could get mad at him?" are attitudes that suppress negative feelings.

Nor releasing negative feelings is a way of holding on to deep hurts, longstanding resentments, and unexpressed grief. No one comes to your aid because they have no idea that you are in trouble. You end up feeling hopeless and helpless, and saying things to yourself like, "What's the use?" Those who experience life this way tend to feel victimized by cancer - that it is a powerful force that they are helpless to overcome. On the other hand, those who see cancer as a challenge to take back power over their own lives are the ones who have the highest survival rate.

Beliefs affect outcomes. Doctors call this the "placebo effect". About 30 percent of the time, those who take an inert sugar pill believing it to be a prescribed drug get better. That is how powerful the mind is. (Ironically, chemotherapy for some forms of cancer works only about 30 percent of the time, the same as for placebo.)

Norman Cousins cured himself of ankylosing spondylitis with laughter and vitamin C. Cousins was awarded an honorary medical degree for this achievement, accepted a post at a university, studied those who survived life threatening illnesses against all odds, and wrote a book entitled, *Head First: The Biology of Hope*. In this book, Norman gives an emotional prescription: "Accept the diagnosis but defy the verdict." Take back your power. Don't believe the medical prognosis. Don't buy into the doom and gloom of other people's beliefs about cancer. Ignore statistics. You have the ability to create your own outcome.

HAZARDS TO AVOID

No matter how strong your immune system may be, there comes a point where it can be overwhelmed. If you sit in the sun long enough, have too many X-rays, or smoke too many cigarettes, you are very likely increasing your risk of developing cancer. The operative word is "likely", because there are exceptions. Some genetically strong individuals can smoke their entire lives and remain cancer-free.

Two daily factors that can overwhelm our immune processes:

Free radicals: radiation (e.g. X-rays, gamma rays, ultra violet, microwaves); tobacco smoke; air pollution; inhalation of toxic chemicals; nitrate/nitrite food preservatives; chronic constipation; polyunsaturated oils.

Heavy metal exposure: aluminum cookware, dental amalgams, contaminated fish, industrial contaminants in the environment.

PREVENTION

A four step program for preventing cancer, or for preventing its recurrence:

1. Reduce exposure to free radical hazards and heavy metals.
2. Avoid junk foods and commercially processed foods in favor of natural whole foods, especially organic.
3. Make olive oil and butter the primary fats in your diet.
4. Supplement with high potency vitamins and antioxidants.

Olive oil is rich in oleic acid, an omega-9 fatty acid that improves immunity at a cellular level. Oleic acid contributes stability to cellular membranes, increasing their resistance to invasion by bacteria, viruses and free radicals. It is for this reason that nature has made oleic acid the predominant fat in mother's milk. Butter provides some oleic acid, plus some short chain saturated fats that the body can de-saturate to form oleic acid, under certain conditions.

If we provide the body with a buffet of all vitamins and minerals in sufficient quantities, the body can select whatever it needs on a given day to strengthen immunity, build strong new cells, and convert proteins into hormones, enzymes and antibodies. For purposes of cancer prevention, an effective supplement program needs to include at least 22 vitamins and minerals, with the following minimum daily amounts of key antioxidants: **Vitamin A** (20,000 IU), **Vitamin C** (4,000 mg.), **Vitamin E** (600 IU), and **Selenium** (200 mcg.). Because of its high content of antioxidants and free radical scavenging agents, the arterial cleansing formula (ACF) described in "Unplug the Arteries" is ideal for this purpose.

An antioxidant is a naturally occurring substance that helps protect cells from the damaging effects of oxygen free radicals, which are highly reactive compounds created during normal cell metabolism. Antioxidants absorb or attach to free radicals, preventing them from attacking normal tissues. If sufficient antioxidants are not available, then the excess free radicals may cause DNA mutations that can lead to cancer.

Green tea, rooibos and yerba mate are excellent sources of dietary antioxidants. So are most berries, including acai, goji, cranberries, blueberries, blackberries, raspberries and strawberries. Apples head the list of antioxidant fruits ("an apple a day keeps the doctor away"). Other fruit sources of antioxidants include peaches, mangos, and melons. Many herbs and spices are rich in antioxidants, including turmeric, cinnamon, rosemary, thyme, oregano, cloves and marjoram.

THYROID FUNCTION

The thyroid gland is the gatekeeper for the rest of the body's metabolic functions. If your thyroid gland is sluggish, the efficiency of all other systems in your body will drop, including your immune processes. In order to prevent cancer, your thyroid needs to function optimally. Your body was designed to work best at a body temperature of 37° Celsius (98.6°

Fahrenheit), and it is the thyroid gland that is responsible for maintaining this temperature.

A simple test: take your temperature three or four times per day between the hours of 10 AM and 5 PM. The average of these readings should be 37°C (98.6°F) or slightly above. If your average daily temperature is below 37 degrees, your thyroid gland is underactive, even if blood tests may suggest otherwise. A blood test indicating underactive thyroid is to be believed. However, a blood test suggesting normal thyroid function is to be doubted. This is because thyroid hormones circulating in the blood may not be reaching the tissues that need them.

There are a number of natural supplements that help to support thyroid function. The most effective of these includes a synergistic blend of iodine, tyrosine, selenium, and cysteine. In some cases, however, natural thyroid support is not enough and prescription thyroid is required. Do whatever it takes to keep your body temperature at a constant 98.6° F during the day.

IODINE

In addition to supporting the thyroid, iodine may help to prevent cancer in other ways. Mainland Japanese consume an average of 13.8 mg. of iodine daily (90 times the RDA), and Japanese women are at extremely low risk for breast, ovarian, and uterine cancer. A number of studies show that women with low iodine intake often have symptoms relating to severe hyperplasia and fibrocystic disease of the breast, which are precancerous lesions that have been corrected by iodine replacement in clinical trials. At least 5 mg. per day of supplemental iodine (from kelp and potassium iodide) is a good investment in your health.

ZINC

Zinc is required in relatively large amounts by the prostate gland, and its deficiency contributes to both BPH (benign prostatic hypertrophy) and to prostatic cancer. Zinc is also a free radical inhibitor, and it helps the body to utilize vitamin A. There is merit in including **zinc** (30 mg.) in one's daily supplements (from gluconate, citrate, or picolinate).

NATURAL CANCER THERAPIES

On a worldwide basis, there may be dozens of effective treatments for cancer that are little known to western civilizations. In cultures that live close to nature, cancer may be statistically infrequent and easily overcome.

One natural remedy that has had a long history of successful use in Canada is Essiac, an herbal combination given to Rene Caisse by a native medicine man. Essiac is a blend of sheep sorrel, burdock root, slippery elm bark, and Indian rhubarb.

Another successful remedy is the Hoxsey formula, a treatment for skin cancer formulated by a veterinarian who observed what horses ate to cure themselves of cancerous growths. The Hoxsey formula consists of select herbs both taken internally and applied to the skin, including red clover, burdock root, licorice root, and some others. Harry Hoxsey, the veterinarian's grandson, wrote a book entitled, *You Don't Have to Die*. The before-and-after photos in this rare book are incredible. Harry, a layman, had a very successful cancer clinic in Texas run by an MD – until that state's government put him out of business by making it illegal for a medical doctor to work for a layperson. That happened over 60 years ago, and there is a cancer clinic in Mexico still successfully using the Hoxsey protocol.

Natural cancer therapies that include low protein diets are to be avoided. Many people with cancer die not from the disease but from starvation induced by too aggressive an attempt to detoxify by restricting protein intake. It is impossible to starve malignant cells without also starving healthy cells.

VITAMIN C

For a time, the medical profession experimented with interferon as a natural cancer remedy. Interferon is a glycoprotein made by the body as an antiviral agent that increases the effectiveness of macrophage immune cells. Interferon is expensive, difficult to harvest, and cannot be duplicated in a laboratory. Ironically, a high intake of vitamin C enables the body to make its own interferon.

There are a number of successful cancer therapies which involve injecting vitamin C intravenously. This an excellent way to deliver high dose vitamin C quickly to cells that are starving for it. Oral vitamin C can only be taken to bowel tolerance, which for many people means that more than 12,000 mg. daily gives them diarrhea or unbearable flatulence. Intravenous vitamin C can be taken in significantly higher amounts.

If you put powdered ascorbic acid crystals (vitamin C) on a plantar's wart and cover with a bandage overnight, after a few of these consecutive treatments, every trace of the wart will be gone. What you will be left with is a crater where the wart used to be. The vitamin C destroys only the wart tissue and leaves the healthy tissue alone. Depending on how deep the wart is, this cure may be quite painful; but it is permanent. The same thing happens if you put ascorbic acid on a small localized skin cancer. Within a few days the cancer will be gone and the healthy tissue intact. If this treatment is attempted on large or deep rooted skin cancers, however, it will need to be quickly followed by surgery to re-join the healthy areas of skin.

Now if vitamin C applied externally can dissolve warts and skin cancers, can vitamin C taken orally reduce the size of internal tumors? Probably, if that vitamin C is in high enough doses and especially if it is accompanied by other high potency antioxidants. Buffered vitamin C (e.g., from calcium ascorbate) is more easily tolerated in high doses than is ascorbic acid.

ANTIOXIDANT THERAPY

Vitamin C is a powerful antioxidant and is even more effective in cancer therapy when combined with other antioxidants, such as beta carotene and selenium. Beta carotene (pro-vitamin A) has been demonstrated to have tumor shrinking properties that vitamin A does not. A low intake of beta carotene is also associated with a high risk for certain cancers.

There was a study that attempted unsuccessfully to discredit beta carotene's ability to shrink tumors. Smokers with lung cancer were given supplementary beta carotene. At the end of the study, some of these smokers' tumors had increased somewhat in size. The most logical explanation for this seeming anomaly is that (a) the subjects in this study were not given enough beta carotene to do the job, too little too late; and (b) smoking probably neutralized some of the benefits of the low dose beta carotene that was given.

It has been estimated that about 300 mcg. of selenium daily can prevent most cancers, whereas typical selenium consumption in North America is about 100 mcg. daily. Selenium is from 200 to 500 times more potent than vitamin E as an antioxidant, and for that reason is very effective when used therapeutically. The body incorporates selenium into glutathione peroxidase, an antioxidant enzyme that detoxifies hydrogen peroxide and fatty acid peroxides. Selenium also assists vitamin E in inhibiting free radicals and protecting tissues from oxidative damage – and it counteracts mercury build-up in the body.

Vitamin E is an antioxidant that protects against free radicals, such as super-oxides, hydroxyl radicals, peroxides and hydro-peroxides. Vitamin E in the amount of 600 IU per day is beneficial to any cancer prevention program. When used therapeutically, however, the action of vitamin E is relatively slow and is unlikely to provide any additional benefit to a program that includes generous amounts of beta carotene, vitamin C and selenium. Once the cancer has been overcome, then vitamin E helps to protect tissues against recurrences.

ALKALINITY

Malignant cells cannot thrive in an environment that is alkaline. For that reason, a number of cancer therapies include going to great lengths to ensure that most food eaten is alkaline. The problem with this approach is that alkaline foods (e.g., vegetables, fruits) are low in protein. Some therapeutic diets for cancer are so low in protein that the patient dies from starvation rather than from the cancer.

To consume a low protein diet during cancer therapy can be self-defeating, because the body needs protein not only to rebuild tissues but also as raw material for antibodies, hormones and enzymes. Good dietary sources of quality protein include eggs, fish, poultry, and soy, preferably all organic.

Balance is important. First step is to eliminate those foods that are highly acid-forming – including sugars, white flour, caffeine, alcohol, and all processed and junk foods. Next step is to make sure that approximately 60 percent of the diet is from plant sources and 40 percent from animal proteins. For total vegetarians (vegans), at least 50 percent of the diet needs to come from either soy or combinations of legumes and grains eaten at the same time (e.g., lentils and rice, beans and corn, hummus on toast, peas and rice, etc.)

If the body has a sufficient intake of electrolyte minerals (e.g., calcium, magnesium, potassium) then it maintains proper pH balance by switching positive and negative mineral ions, as needed. For most adults who eat sensibly, daily supplements that include **calcium** (800 mg.), **magnesium** (500 mg.), and **potassium** (400 mg.) are enough to maintain alkalinity of blood, saliva and urine.

DETOXIFICATION

When immune and eliminative systems are weak or overburdened, the body accumulates foreign debris and metabolic waste products that it would otherwise have disposed of through urine, the bowels, the skin or even exhaling. Cells become strangled in their own waste and become unable to accept the nutrients they need for their thriving.

Many who have cancer are in need of some form of detoxification. Accumulated heavy metals may be contributing to the cancer, and/or excess cellular waste products may be a symptom of the low immune and low thyroid functions which invited the cancer.

Fasting, the total elimination of all solid food is a popular way to let the body get on with its housecleaning, so to speak, by giving it a vacation from having to digest food. However, this is an extreme measure that can be carried too far. Some have the mistaken belief that fasting is a way to "starve" the cancer. You cannot do that without also starving the rest of the body. Many cancer patients die from malnutrition and not from the disease.

Juice fasting for one to three days only is a safer alternative. In this modified fast, one abstains from solid food but consumes freshly juiced lemons, beets, carrots, radishes, and other fruits and vegetables according to their reputed cleansing properties. Diabetics should never fast, nor should anyone whose body is a depleted or emaciated state.

Even short term juice fasting may not be necessary if one is on high dose antioxidant therapy. Large amounts of vitamin C, in particular, perk up the immune and eliminative systems, enabling the body to catch up on its housecleaning.

ALLERGIES

Some forms of cancer may be caused by allergies; and when the allergens are avoided, the immune system becomes empowered to dispose of the malignant cells. An allergy is an acquired, abnormal immune response.

Most healthy people have immune systems that are strong enough to deal with mild or moderate exposure to, say, petrochemicals and heavy metals. But if one acquires an allergy to these substances, then the immune system becomes paralyzed to deal with them. As the petrochemicals or heavy metals advance, the immune system retreats, so to speak; and tumors can be the result.

To correct an allergy can be easily done with homeopathy. A homeopathic remedy is a micro dilution of the substance that is causing the harm. Taking this remedy orally stimulates the immune system to overcome the cause. For example, a 30C dilution of petroleum taken under the tongue for two months enables the body to overcome its allergy to petrochemicals – and by so doing empowers the immune system to deal with both the petrochemicals and the cancer.

A 30C homeopathic is so dilute that there are no molecules of any substance left in it. No molecules means no side effects. This remedy simply carries the energetic imprint of, say, petroleum – which stimulates the immune system to deal with the invader.

Everyone with cancer is well advised to take the following two remedies, each to be taken 10 drops under the tongue three times daily, between meals: (1) **Petroleum** 30 C, and (2) a 30 C combination of **Aluminium, Cadmium, Lead, Mercury** and **Nickel.** Two months is long enough on these homeopathics to correct allergies. If these remedies do not provide any perceived benefit in two months, it means that petroleum and heavy metals were not contributing to the cancer.

In some cases, the above 30C remedies may be a key factor in overcoming the cancer. In others, they will be an adjunct to help the body detoxify itself. Even in cases where homeopathy may be of no benefit, there is no down side. It is something that is safe and inexpensive to try, rather like a form of insurance.

A CANCER FORMULA

"It is a false idea that the benefits of chemotherapy are blunted if one takes vitamin A, vitamin C and/or selenium along with the chemo. The opposite is true. The latest evidence is that nutrients such as these make conventional cancer treatments work better." - Ralph W. Moss, "Antioxicants Against Cancer"

There are a number of effective nutritional therapies for cancer. The following is one that has a 22-year history of successful use. Its high level of beta carotene and antioxidants help not only to shrink tumors, but also to prevent hair loss and to protect healthy tissue from the harmful effects of chemotherapy. Best taken in divided amounts with meals:

Vitamin A (as beta carotene)	110,000 I.U.
Vitamin C (ascorbic acid/ca. ascorbate	7,000 mg.
Niacin	15 mg.
Calcium (carbonate/ascorbate)	1,750 mg.
Iodine (potassium iodide)	6,000 mcg.
DL-Methionine	30 mg.
Selenium	250 mcg.
Trimethylglycine	60 mg.

The ingredients in the above formula function as antioxidants, free radical scavengers, and immune builders. Some people may develop a yellowish tint to their skin because of the high amount of beta carotene in this formula. This discoloration is entirely safe, *if* due to beta carotene – and this needs to be distinguished from jaundice. In jaundice the whites of the eyes also turn yellow. In beta carotene discoloration, the whites of the eyes remain white.

Users of this cancer formula have reported complete remission of prostate cancer, breast cancer, brain tumors, lymphoma, and spinal cancer. There seems to be a 50:50 split between who used only the nutritional approach and who used it as an adjunct to chemotherapy and radiation.

My mother is one of many who can attest to the effectiveness of the above formula. At age 75, she took it as an adjunct to the surgery and chemotherapy prescribed for her colon cancer. She came through the experience with flying colors, never losing a single hair from her head. That was 20 years ago, and her cancer has never returned.

Beta-carotene prevents tissue damage by trapping organic free radicals. People with the highest intakes or blood levels of beta-carotene have a 20 to 40 percent lower risk of cancer than those with the lowest intakes or blood levels. Controlled studies have reported its efficacy in reversing precancerous lesions.

Vitamin C intake and plasma/serum levels of vitamin C are both inversely associated with cancer risk. The literature suggests that supplementation with vitamin C may reduce the risk of cancer at several sites. Not only does supplemental vitamin C kill tumor cells, but it also stimulates the host's immune system against residual tumor cells. Vitamin C inhibits the carcinogenic nitrosamines and nitrosamides formed from dietary nitrites and nitrates. High levels of vitamin C enhances the effects of chemotherapy and radiation therapy.

DL-methionine is an amino acid that counteracts free radical processes. It is used in the prevention and treatment of certain types of liver damage and is also a methyl donor used in anti-fatigue supplements.

Selenium status is inversely related to cancer risk. and serum selenium is an excellent predictor of the subsequent development of cancer. Selenium supplementation is associated with reduction in total cancer mortality, total cancer incidence, and the incidences of lung, colorectal, and prostate cancers. Selenium supplementation may reduce tissue damage from chemotherapy.

Glutathione is a tri-peptide found in a variety of foods. It may function as an anti-carcinogen by acting as an antioxidant and by binding with cellular mutagens. Its dietary intake may be inversely associated with oral and pharyngeal cancer risk. Total plasma levels of glutathione are markedly decreased in many types of cancer. Supplementation with glutathione may inhibit carcinogenesis.

Trimethylglycine is a natural substance that is widely distributed in plants and animals. It enhances both humoral and cell mediated immune responses.

ADAPTOGENS

Adaptogens are natural substance that help the body adapt to stress. The herbal adaptogens that are of most benefit as an adjunct to every kind of cancer therapy are those which improve the alkalinity of bodily tissues – because malignant cells cannot thrive in an alkaline environment. Examples of such alkalizing adaptogens include **Goji fruit** (*Lycium barbarum*), **Red Clover** (*Trifolium pratense*), and **Fo Ti** (*Polygonum multiflorum*),

CATARACTS

A cataract is a whitening opacity of the normally transparent lens (and/or lens capsule) of the eye, resulting from damage to the protein structure of the lens, usually by free radicalsw. Cataracts commonly accompany aging and can be precipitated by infection, injury, side reactions to drugs, diabetic complications, cigarette smoking, and overexposure to radiation (including ultraviolet rays from the sun). In cataract formation, the body's normal protective mechanisms are unable to prevent damage from free radicals.

The lens of the eye has the highest protein content (35 percent) of any tissue of the body. It also requires a 20 times greater concentration of vitamin C than is in the blood. The lens is especially vulnerable because it is not nourished directly from the bloodstream. It has to receive the nutrients it needs indirectly, from adjacent tissues. Low protein diets increase the risk for cataracts significantly.

There is a nutritional way to halt the progression of cataracts, and also to reverse those which are not too far advanced. This method can also be of benefit to other conditions of the eye, such as macular degeneration. It protects the lens of the eye from free radical damage in two ways: (1) by providing five nutritional antioxidants (vitamin C, vitamin E, selenium, beta carotene, glutathione), and (2) by supplying the raw materials from which the body makes five enzymatic antioxidants (superoxide dismustase, catalase, glutathione peroxidase, glutathione reductase).

Beta carotene acts as a filter, protecting against light-induced damage to the fiber portion of the lens. The blood level of beta-carotene is inversely associated with cataract risk. Those with serum levels of beta-carotene in the lowest third of distribution have a threefold risk of senile cataracts.

Vitamin E intake and vitamin E blood levels are both inversely related to the risk of cataracts. Vitamin E protects the lens against free radical damage – and may offer protection against the destructive effects of diabetes. The levels of both superoxide dismutase and glutathione reductase decrease as a result of vitamin E deficiency.

Vitamin C intake and vitamin C blood levels are both inversely correlated with cataract risk. Vitamin C protects against ultraviolet light-induced cataracts. In clinical trials, from 60 to 90 percent of patients with incipient senile cataracts had significant visual improvement following supplementation with vitamin C.

Riboflavin (vitamin B-2) deficiency is associated with the risk of pre-senile and senile cataracts. A riboflavin deficiency may promote cataract formation by interfering with glutathione reductase activity. In clinical trials there has been dramatic improvement in patients with fully developed cataracts after supplementation with riboflavin. A high lactose intake may promote the development of cataracts by causing a riboflavin deficiency.

Methonine and **cysteine** are rate limiting amino acids in the body's synthesis of glutathione. Increasing the intake of methionine and cysteine may help to prevent cataract formation by retarding the age-related decline in glutathione levels.

Selenium is required by the enzymatic antioxidant, glutathione peroxidase, for its functioning. Blood levels of selenium appear to be reduced in patients with senile cataracts and are positively correlated with aqueous humor levels of erythrocyte glutathione peroxidase. Patients with senile cataracts may have reduced selenium levels in the aqueous humor. The selenium concentration of cataractous lenses may be only 15 percent of normal.

Glutathione is the antioxidant substrate for two important antioxidant enzymes, glutathione peroxidase and glutathione reductase. Whereas glutathione levels decrease gradually in normal lenses with advancing age, cataractous lenses contain only about one-tenth as much glutathione. As glutathione levels fall, lens oxidation increases. Glutathione levels are positively correlated with the activity of superoxide dismutase in the cataractous lens.

ANTI-CATARACT FORMULA

Daily supplementation with a broad spectrum of nutrients that includes the following has a 30-year history of successfully halting, reducing, and reversing cataracts. By providing a broad spectrum of high potency nutrients required by the eye, this formula also assists the body in overcoming other degenerative eye conditions that have a nutritional cause – including macular degeneration, vitamin A and riboflavin deficiencies, and discoloration of the whites of the eyes.

Vitamin A	30,000 I.U.
Beta-Carotene (pro-vitamin A)	50,000 I.U.
Vitamin E	400 I.U.
Vitamin C (ascorbic acid)	3,000 mg.
Vitamin B-2 (riboflavin)	100 mg.
Selenium	200 mcg.
DL-Methionine	150 mg.
L-Cysteine	200 mg.
L-Glutamine	200 mg.
Glycine	50 mg.
Glutathione	30 mg.

Lutein (xanthophyll) is an antioxidant carotenoid that protects eye tissue. The above formula is so powerful in antioxidant and beta carotene activity, however, that adding lutein to it would not provide any additional benefit. Lutein is found in green leafy vegetables, spinach, kale, yellow carrots, and eggs. During World War II, pilots received top priority for rationed eggs. The beta carotene and lutein content of eggs was probably responsible for maintaining their night vision.

Although the above formula was designed for reversing cataracts, for which purpose it is extremely effective, it is also of considerable benefit for every eye condition that is caused by nutritional deficiency. Some people's vision has improved to the extent that they no longer require glasses for driving. A number of optometrists have observed cellular regeneration that is otherwise not possible – especially in correcting dry eye syndrome, a condition their profession believes to be permanent. There have also been a number of reports that this formula has significantly improved macular degeneration, a condition that limits one's ability to visualize fine details.

EYE EXERCISES

The above formula cannot restore vision loss that is caused by atrophying eye muscles. Eye exercises, however, can do that.

The focal length of the eye is the distance between the lens and the retina (usually about 1.7 cm.). What keeps this distance a constant is the consistently round shape of the eyeball, which is maintained by the extraocular muscles. As these muscles lose their tone, the focal length of the eye changes – with the result that the image projected onto the retina becomes slightly blurred. That is when eyeglasses are prescribed, to modify the image coming through the lens to compensate for the changed focal length. As the eye muscles gradually deteriorate, stronger and stronger eyeglasses are required.

Eye muscles are like other muscles: they need regular exercise. The following are exercises that strengthen and tone the extraocular muscles for the sole purpose of restoring focal length. I call them "eye pushups".

Before starting on eye pushups, I had astigmatism in my right eye and had to wear prescription bifocals for everything I did, all day long. The reading portion of these lens averaged 3.25 diopters. After six months of eye pushups, I now wear standard glasses only for reading, with lenses of 1.50 diopters – and my vision is still improving. If the astigmatism is still there, it is of no consequence.

Here is how to do eye pushups. Hold the eraser end of a pencil upwards, about the same distance from your face as you would hold a book. Focus on some distant point within the room or looking out the window. Quickly shift your vision to the end of the pencil, and hold that focus just long enough to say you did – then just as quickly shift your focus back to the distant point. Do this for 22 repetitions. Repeat the exercise five times daily. Persistence pays off.

PROSTATE ENLARGEMENT

The prostate is a walnut-sized, donut-shaped gland below the bladder that surrounds the male urethra. It secretes a milky, alkaline fluid that increases sperm motility and lubricates the urethra to prevent infection. Enlargement of the prostate is common, especially after middle age. This condition is known as benign prostatic hyperplasia (BPH). It results in urethral obstruction that impedes urination.

Symptoms of BPH include: frequent need to urinate, reduced force and speed of urination, difficulty urinating (starting, burning), urinate more than twice during the night, unable to empty bladder completely, back pains associated with urinary difficulties, lost or diminished sex drive, and/or discomfort or dull aching in the perineal area (between scrotum and anus). [Warning: *If you have any of the above symptoms, get a medical diagnosis. Prostate cancer, the second leading cause of death in men, has similar symptoms.*]

With age, levels of the male sex hormone, testosterone, decrease but estrogen levels increase. The lower level of testosterone within the prostate gland compensates by increasing in concentration and converting to a more potent form, dihydrotestosterone (DHT). In BPH, it is thought that excess estrogen is the key factor that inhibits the elimination of DHT.

BPH affects over 50 percent of men during their lifetime. Its frequency increases with age, from under 10 percent at age 30 to over 90 percent in men over 85 years of age. If left untreated, BPH eventually results in complete retention of urine and kidney damage. Fortunately, nutritional methods can reverse this condition, which is caused by a lack of specific nutrients required by the prostate for its optimal functioning.

The prostate gland has the highest concentration of zinc of any organ or tissue in the body. It also has very high requirements for three amino acids: glycine, alanine and glutamic acid.

Zinc normally binds to the cells of the prostate; however, its ability to do so is reduced during BPH. Although prostatic and blood levels of zine may be normal, the prostatic cells may actually be zinc deprived. Zinc supplementation inhibits the activity of 5-alpha-reductase, the enzyme that converts testosterone to DHT. Zinc inhibits the pituitary's secretion of prolactin, a hormone that increases the uptake of testosterone by the prostate.

Glycine, alanine and **glutamic acid** are amino acids found in large amounts in prostate tissue. Supplements of these three have both shrink the prostate and relieve symptoms of BPH – including nighttime urination, urinary frequency, and delayed urination.

Muscular weakness also contributes to BPH. The prostate muscles need to be exercised, and this can be done by applying gentle finger pressure to the perineum (point midway between scrotum and anus). Hold for two seconds, relax, then repeat five or six times more. Do this twice daily.

PROSTATE SUPPORT

Daily supplementation with the following nutrients has a 25-year history of successfully reducing benign prostatic hyperplasia: **zinc** (75 mg.), **L-alanine** (40 mg.), **glycine** (30 mg.), **glutamic acid** (30 mg.), and **prostate substance** (80 mg.). If some of the above are not available, **saw palmetto** and **pumpkin seed oil** may be able to help. The zinc, however, is mandatory.

CANDIDIASIS

Candidiasis refers to an overgrowth of the fungus, *Candida albicans*. The candida organism is a normal inhabitant of our intestinal tract. Under certain conditions, however, candida proliferates out of control, forcing itself into the intestinal lining, where it destroys cells in the microvilli, passes into the bloodstream and invades tissues where it does not belong (systemic candidiasis). The destruction of cells in the microvilli reduce the permeability of the small intestine, thus creating what is commonly known as a "leaky gut".

Symptoms of candidiasis can include the following:

☐ cravings for sugars, bread or alcohol.
☐ indigestion/discomfort after eating fruits or sweets.
☐ severe reactions to perfumes, tobacco, chemicals.
☐ intolerance to alcohol.
☐ hypersensitivity to certain foods.
☐ diarrhea or constipation.
☐ rectal itching or bladder infections.
☐ coated or sore tongue.
☐ chronic sore or scratchy throat, oral thrush.
☐ feel bad all over, without apparent cause.
☐ feeling of being in a mental fog, "spaciness."
☐ hives, psoriasis or skin rash.
☐ anxiety or depression.
☐ tiredness, feelings of being "drained."
☐ athlete's foot, toenail or fingernail fungus.
☐ allergy or sensitivity to airborne molds.
☐ allergy or sensitivity to moldy or fermented foods.

- [ ] premenstrual tension, menstrual cramps.
- [ ] vaginal discharge, burning, itching.
- [ ] endometriosis, uterine fibroids.
- [ ] prostate problems, impotence.
- [ ] itching of penis or groin.

Many people with candidiasis have been heavy users of broad-spectrum antibiotics, steroid drugs, birth control pills, or alcohol. These drugs destroy the beneficial microflora in the intestines that are the natural antagonists of *C. albicans*. They need to be avoided, as much as possible.

Most candida programs are not very effective. This is because they do nothing for the cause of the problem. Because *Candida albicans* is a normal inhabitant of the intestinal tract, it cannot be starved out of the body. What allows candida to overpopulate is a weak immune system. The only way to reduce the candida population to normal levels is to restore that immunity.

Virtually everyone with candidiasis has acquired an allergy to the candida organism. This allergy paralyzes the immune processes that would normally keep the candida in check. This allergy can be reversed, however, simply by taking a homeopathic 30C dilution of *Candida albicans* - 10 drops under the tongue three times daily, between meals. If the only thing you do for candidiasis is to take this homeopathic remedy every day for two months, the candida population will likely be back to normal levels within six months. This time frame can be shortened considerably by also taking garlic and caprylic acid (anti-fungal agents) and *Lactobacillus acidophilus* (or similar probiotic).

If the candidiasis is systemic (i.e., in the bloodstream), then oregano oil will likely be of immediate benefit. Oil of oregano is very potent. It needs to be taken two to three drops under the tongue, twice daily, between meals and at least 30 minutes after taking the homeopathic remedy.

If the candida allergy is **not** corrected, then the strictest diet will not bring lasting results. If the allergy **is** corrected, then the candida control diet does not have to be harsh. The important things to eliminate are alcohol and concentrated sugars/sweets of all kinds, including fruit juices and dried fruits. (One piece of whole fruit per day is usually not a problem.) It is sometimes helpful also to eliminate fermented foods (e.g., vinegar, pickles, sauerkraut, tempeh, miso, tofu). With the homeopathic control program, it is not necessary to eliminate foods containing yeasts (e.g., baker's, brewer's, torula) – unless the person also has allergies to those specific yeasts.

Although *Candida albicans* is a natural inhabitant of the digestive tract, it does **not** belong in the bloodstream. It can arrive there only by passing through an intestinal wall that is more permeable that it ought to be. Therefore, wherever systemic candidiasis is found, a leaky gut will also require attention.

LEAKY GUT

If the small intestine becomes more permeable than it is supposed to be (i.e., "leaky"), it allows abnormally large food molecules to enter the bloodstream. These incompletely digested molecules stimulate allergic/immune responses both in the intestinal wall and elsewhere in the body. In additional to gastrointestinal complaints, symptoms may be produced in the skin (hives or eczema), joints (arthritis), lungs (asthma), or almost anywhere else.

When the small intestine loses its filtration abilities (intestinal impermeability), it both absorbs what it should not and does not absorb what it should. Vitamin B-12 and the fat soluble vitamins (A, D, E and K) pass through the leaky gut with great difficulty, often leaving the individual deficient in these vital nutrients.

The healthy intestinal wall absorbs only proteins that have been broken down into single amino acids or into tiny molecules consisting of two or three amino acids (dipeptides, tripeptides). The small intestine is also a first line in our immune defence. Not only does it prevent harmful microbes and toxic substances from entering the bloodstream, it also produces an antibody (secretory IgA) that neutralizes invaders and prevents them from attaching to membranes.

A leaky gut allows not only oversize protein molecules to enter the bloodstream but also bacteria, viruses, fungi and parasites. When this happens, the body reacts with alarm. The immune system builds IgG antibodies to these foreign molecules. Many diverse allergic and auto-immune reactions may follow. Chronic fatigue is common, as it is a symptom of a body constantly struggling with a perpetual threat. Almost every meal creates systemic stress for the body that has a leaky gut. The longer the body is under siege in this way, the less able it is to produce the antibodies and hormones it needs.

The leaky gut both absorbs what it should not and does not absorb what it should. Its ability to absorb certain vitamins (e.g., A, D, E, B-12, folic acid) and minerals (e.g., copper, iron, magnesium, selenium, zinc) is greatly impaired. Thus, a person with this syndrome may have significant deficiencies of several key nutrients in spite of an adequate intake of them. Supplementing with generous amounts of these factors can both compensate for their poor absorption and also speed the healing process.

A laboratory test which reveals low IgG antibodies is usually indicative of leaky gut. The presence of either parasites or candida in the bloodstream is another indicator of a leaky gut. Symptoms of a leaky gut can include:

☐ constipation and/or diarrhea.
☐ abdominal pain or bloating.
☐ indigestion or flatulence.
☐ mucus or blood in stools.
☐ chronic joint or muscle pains.
☐ chronic fatigue, tiredness.
☐ fuzzy thinking.
☐ confusion, poor memory.
☐ mood swings.
☐ poor exercise tolerance.
☐ weak immunity.
☐ shortness of breath.
☐ skin rashes, hives, eczema.
☐ asthma, bronchitis, respiratory infections.
☐ sinus or nasal congestion.
☐ food allergies/intolerances.
☐ alcohol consumption makes one feel sick.

A leaky gut may be caused by gluten intolerance (celiac disease), non-steroidal anti-inflammatory drugs (NSAIDs), alcohol, intestinal parasites, food sensitivities, candidiasis, or by continually overloading a sluggish digestive system with far more food than it can handle. All of the contributing factors need to be identified and eliminated in order to allow the intestinal wall to repair itself.

Alcohol is absorbed directly into the blood from the stomach and upper small intestine. On its way through, it destroys cells in the stomach and intestinal linings. Consuming alcohol with food helps to minimize this damage. A healthy body can metabolize small amounts of alcohol; however, anyone with a suspected leaky guy would be wise to avoid alcohol entirely.

Candidiasis refers to an overgrowth of the fungus, *Candida albicans* in the gut that can either create a leaky gut or pass through one that has previously been formed from other causes. Most people with candidiasis have been heavy users of broad-spectrum antibiotics, steroid drugs, or birth control pills. These drugs destroy the beneficial microflora in the intestines that are the natural antagonists of *C. albicans*.

Intestinal parasites are more common than many people realize. Supplementing with a broad spectrum digestive aid providing hydrochloric acid and bile helps to sterilize them from the intestines. *L. acidophilus* (or similar probiotic) can displace parasites in the gut. Herbs such as garlic, grapefruit seed extract, pumpkin seed, wormwood, and black walnut hulls can kill intestinal parasites.

Food allergies always attack a particular organ or structure in the body. If the target organ happens to be the small intestine, then its lining could be damaged. Thus, hidden food allergies may contribute to the development of a leaky gut.

DIGESTIVE WEAKNESSES

Two digestive weaknesses contribute to the leaky gut syndrome: (1) an inability to break down proteins into their smallest components, and (2) deterioration of the intestinal lining. First, if there were no oversize protein molecules, they would never end up in the bloodstream. Secondly, if the intestinal wall had ideal permeability, it would not allow oversized polypeptides to pass through.

Sometimes the intestinal lining becomes so weakened that it has difficulty handling most solid foods, especially those containing any appreciable amount of protein or starch. In such cases it needs a complete rest in order to recover. The medical option would be parenteral nutrition, in which all food is taken intravenously, giving the small intestine nothing to do except heal itself. Fortunately, there is a less extreme approach that can work as well. It relies on getting one's nutritional requirements from generous amounts of pre-digested (hydrolyzed) protein, fruits, non-starchy vegetables, and olive oil.

REPAIR THE INTESTINAL LINING

The surface microvilli in the small intestine are highly regenerative. If given a total rest from everything that irritates them, individual microvilli can repair themselves within four to five days. If damage is extensive there will be deeper tears in the intestinal wall, and healing will take much longer – and healing of the gut needs to be total in order for the body's overall health to be restored.

We would not expect a cut on our skin to heal if we continually rubbed it with abrasives. So it is with the delicate internal "skin" that lines our intestinal tract. If, however, we diligently identify and eliminate all of the substances that are irritating it, it will heal itself. Healing supplements (e.g., vitamins A, C and E) can aid in this self-repairing process – if and only if all of the intestinal irritants are removed from the diet.

The ideal diet for repairing the leaky gut is one that is as hypoallergenic as possible. Ideally, it should eliminate all milk products, all gluten-containing grains, all sugars, all refined flour products, all high-fat foods, all alcohol, plus all other foods that individual experience has shown to cause any manner of gastrointestinal distress, plus all other foods to which one is known to be allergic (or is suspected of being allergic).

A leaky gut cannot process large protein molecules, so these are to be avoided. Starches and disaccharide sugars (sucrose, lactose) are also to be avoided because a damaged intestinal wall is unable to produce the final enzymes needed to break them down. Incompletely digested starches and sugars remain in the gut, fermenting and feeding pathogenic bacteria, candida and other microbes that continue to attack the intestinal wall.

The form of sugar that is most compatible with healing a leaky gut is fructose (fruit sugar). Fructose is a monosaccharide, a simple sugar that is readily absorbed through the intestinal wall without requiring any action by digestive enzymes. Fructose has the same chemical formula as glucose, but its molecule twists in the opposite direction. Before the body can use fructose, the liver has to change it into glucose, a conversion that takes about 22 minutes. Thus fructose is not released into the bloodstream quite as quickly as glucose.

FOODS TO AVOID

In order to heal the leaky gut it is necessary to eliminate *all* of the following:

- milk products: butter, buttermilk, cheese, cottage cheese, ice cream, ice milk, kefir, milk, quark, yogurt.
- grains: amaranth, barley, buckwheat, bulgur, corn, kamut, millet, oats, quinoa, rice, rye, semolina, spelt, triticale, wheat, wild rice.
- legumes: peas, beans, lentils, chickpeas, soy/tofu, etc.
- starchy vegetables: beets, carrots, parsnips, potatoes, pumpkin, winter squash, sweet potatoes, turnip, yams.
- high glycemic fruits: banana, dried fruits, fruit juices.
- sugars: brown sugar, cane juice, corn syrup, Demerara sugar, dextri-maltose, dextrose, glucose, icing sugar, malto-dextrin, maltose, maple sugar, molasses, raw sugar, rice syrup, sucrose, table sugar, turbinado sugar, white sugar.
- alcoholic beverages.
- nuts and seeds.

THE DIET: PHASE 1

Phase I of the diet to heal the leaky gut consists of only the following foods:

- hydrolyzed (pre-digested) protein powder blended with water and fresh fruit (*not* fruit juice) to make a "smoothie."
- fresh, whole fruits, of as wide a variety as possible, preferably organic, and in any reasonable quantity to satisfy hunger – e.g., apples, apricots, berries (all kinds), cantaloupe, cherries, fresh currants, fresh figs, grapefruit, grapes, guava, honeydew melon, kiwi, lemons, limes, mangoes, nectarines, oranges, papaya, passion fruit, peaches, pears, persimmon, pineapple, plums, pomegranate, star fruit, tangerine, watermelon.
- fresh, non-starchy vegetables, preferably organic, and in any reasonable quantity to satisfy hunger – e.g., alfalfa sprouts, artichokes, asparagus, bamboo shoots, bean sprouts, beet greens, bell peppers, bok choi, broccoli, Brussels sprouts, cabbage, cauliflower, celery, chicory greens, chives, cilantro, clove sprouts, collard greens, crookneck squash, cucumber, daikon, dandelion

greens, eggplant, endive, escarole, fennel, garlic, green beans, horseradish, iceberg lettuce, jicima, kale, kohlrabi, leeks, okra, onions, radish, romaine lettuce, mustard greens, parsley, pickles, sauerkraut, scallions, spaghetti squash, spinach, summer squash, Swiss chard, tomatillo, tomatoes, turnip greens, watercress, wax beans, yellow beans, zucchini.

- organic <u>olive oil</u>, 2 to 3 tablespoonsful per day, taken at the same time as the non-starchy vegetables (e.g., as a salad dressing).
- <u>honey</u> (a source of fructose), 1 tablespoon per day, between meals or with fruits.
- <u>beverages</u>: purified water, decaffeinated teas, decaffeinated coffee.
- <u>condiments</u>: lemon juice, lime juice, vinegar.

All of the above are to be consumed <u>according to the following guidelines</u>:

- Have the largest meal of the day at noon.
- Wait 3 hours after any meal that contains olive oil before consuming anything else.
- Wait 30 minutes after fruit or hydrolyzed protein shakes before consuming a meal that contains olive oil.

As long as the above timing guidelines are followed, fresh fruit or veggies (without oil) may be consumed as a separate snack as often as desired throughout the day.

THE DIET: PHASE 2

The dietary guidelines are the same as for Phase 1, except that nuts (without skins, blanched), seeds, eggs, fish and/or poultry may be consumed (again, preferably organic). Every time animal protein is eaten however, an appropriate number of digestive enzyme tablets is to be taken. All appropriate vitamin-mineral supplements are also to be taken during this phase. Herbs and spices can also be added back. Hydrolyzed protein may be combined with fruits or vegetables as desired, but not with fruit juice.

LENGTH OF TREATMENT

The intestinal healing program consists of two parts, each of which lasts for three weeks.

Phase 1 includes only those foods on the above "acceptable" list. Homeopathic remedies may also be taken, but no vitamin, mineral, glandular or herbal supplements of any kind – also no spices and no herbal teas.

Phase 2 follows the same guidelines, except that protein foods may be added – such as eggs, fish, poultry, or fermented soy (miso, tempeh, or tofu only). Every time protein is eaten, an appropriate amount of a suitable digestive enzyme formula is also to be taken. All vitamin-mineral and amino acid supplements appropriate to the individual's needs are also to be taken during this phase. Dietary proteins may be combined with the non-starchy vegetables and with the olive oil.

The complete program consists of three weeks on Phase 1, followed by 3 weeks on Phase 2, followed by three weeks on Phase 1 ... and so on ... for up to six months to heal the most stubborn cases. It is a strict and challenging program to follow, but it is what the small intestine needs in order to do its own healing. If at any time the program should cause undue hardship, then modify it – either by adding particular supplements to Phase 1, or by shortening the time spent on Part 1 and lengthening the time spent on Phase 2. Dairy products, grains, legumes, starches and di-saccharide sugars are the enemies of intestinal healing. If you must consume any of them during the program, do so infrequently. Your body can more easily handle a large quantity consumed once in a while than it can small amounts eaten every day.

The leaky gut both absorbs what it should not and does not absorb what it should. Its ability to absorb essential fatty acids, certain vitamins (e.g., A, D, E, B-12, folic acid) and certain minerals (e.g., copper, iron, magnesium, selenium, zinc) is greatly impaired. Thus, a person with this syndrome may have significant deficiencies of several key nutrients in spite of an adequate intake of them. Supplementing with generous amounts of these factors can both compensate for their poor absorption and speed the healing process.

AUTOIMMUNE DISORDERS

Autoimmune disorders include such diverse conditions as ankylosing spondylitis, Crohn's disease, fibromyalgia, glomerulonephritis, hemolytic anemia, lupus erythematosus, multiple sclerosis, myasthenia gravis, myopathy, neuromuscular degeneration, polymyalgia rheumatica, Raynaud's syndrome, rheumatoid arthritis, scleroderma, Scorgen's syndrome, chronic thyroiditis, Grave's disease, Creutzfeld-Jacob disease, ulcerative colitis, vasculitis, and vitiligo. What all of these conditions have in common is that the body attacks its own tissues. How they differ is in which tissues are attacked. Scientists know how this happens, but not why. A number of theories have been proposed, none of which give the full picture

Antigens are what trigger immune responses. An antigen is any substance that causes the body to produce antibodies against it. Each antibody is specifically produced by the immune system to match an antigen after immune cells have come into contact with it. The antibody "matches" the antigen in the sense that it can bind to it. In most cases, an antibody can bind to only one specific antigen. In some instances, however, antibodies may bind to more than one antigen – in a phenomenon called "cross-reactivity".

The cross-reactivity between natural latex rubber and some fruits (e.g., avocado, kiwi, banana) is well known. Someone who has an allergic reaction to inhaled latex molecules is likely to have the same reaction to eating a banana. This is because antibodies produced to match one structure necessarily match the same structure if it happens to be found in unrelated proteins from divergent sources or other species.

Our immune system recognizes particular antigen structures as foreign without regard to the origin of these molecules. If a foreign protein fragment finds its way into the blood (i.e., through a leaky gut), then the antibodies produced to match the invader will also match identical protein structures wherever they may be found in the host's body. This is clearly what happened in mad cow's disease (BSE).

MAD COW'S DISEASE

The outbreak of mad cow's disease [*bovine spongiform encephalopathy (BSE)*] and the fear that it could spread to humans peaked my curiosity. What we were being told about this condition made no sense, so I did my own analysis and concluded that BSE is (or was) an artificially induced autoimmune disorder.

The most telling piece of evidence is that the only cattle affected by BSE were those who were fed ground sheep's brains mixed in with their feed. This was commercially motivated – to sell a by-product of slaughtering sheep that would increase the protein quality of the bovine diet. Science, however, was totally ignored. Cattle are herbivores (total vegetarians) whose digestive systems are incapable of breaking down and assimilating animal proteins. Partially digested bits of sheep's brains found their way into the blood of the cattle, whose immune systems made antibodies to these foreign proteins. The proteins in sheep's brain cells, however, are identical to the proteins in cattle's brain cells, so the antibodies designed to get rid of the foreign invader also attacked the host's brain cells.

BSE never spread from one herd to another, nor from one animal to another. It was confined exclusively to those animals that had consumed sheep's brains. No infective agent was ever found – no bacteria, no virus, no parasite, no fungus - nothing that could have spread the disease.

What scientists did find in the blood and brains of the affected cattle were tiny protein fragments called "prions" – which were one of the effects of the disease rather than its cause. Prions are leftover protein fragments that the overwhelmed antibodies were unable to clear away.

There was a false fear that BSE could jump the species barrier and affect humans. This never happened, nor could it. Creutzfeldt-Jakob disease (CJD) in humans is similar to BSE in that both diseases result from antibodies attacking the brain and leaving behind prions. Both are autoimmune disorders. Neither is communicable. It would be interesting to find out how many people with CJD (and a leaky gut) had been eating monkey brains (a Chinese and Indonesian delicacy).

LEAKY GUT

A leaky gut may contribute to some autoimmune disorders. If the small intestine becomes more permeable than it is supposed to be (i.e., "leaky"), it allows abnormally large protein molecules to enter the bloodstream. When this happens, the body reacts with alarm and makes antibodies to these foreign molecules. Unfortunately, if the amino acid configuration in these invaders is identical to protein structures in certain bodily tissues, the antibodies attack those host tissues also.

Weak digestion and a leaky gut allow into the blood partially digested proteins from meat (as an example) consumed at a meal. Antibodies to these muscle proteins in the blood could also attack the person's muscles, creating autoimmune myositis (inflammation of voluntary muscle tissue). Antibodies to cartilage molecules in the blood could similarly create autoimmune chondritis (inflammation of cartilage). Liver cells in the blood might create autoimmune hepatitis … and so on. So far so good.

Now here is where it gets tricky. Cross-reactivity tells us that the bodily cell being attacked could be as different from the antigen in the blood as latex rubber is to a banana. The antibody has to match only a small part of the structure of two completely unrelated proteins for cross-reactivity to occur. The implication is that any partially digested protein molecule in the blood could potentially trigger any autoimmune disorder in a uniquely sensitive person.

A POSSIBLE CAUSE

Many autoimmune disorders may have causes that are as yet unknown. What I am proposing is a leaky gut theory of autoimmunity that may explain some of them. To find out to what extent this theory applies can only be done on a person by person basis. A leaky gut should be suspect in anyone suffering from autoimmunity who also has a history of factors that damage the intestinal lining – including gluten intolerance, non-steroidal ant-inflammatory (NSAID) drug use, excessive alcohol intake, candidiasis, and food allergies.

Gluten tolerance (celiac disease) is a strong possibility. I know a number of celiac patients who later developed fibromyalgia. The celiac intestine characteristically has many microvilli broken off, leaving gaping holes in this important filter.

Non-steroidal anti-inflammatory drugs (e.g., aspirin, ibuprofen) are given to reduce inflammation and pain. It is ironic that NSAIDs can also create inflammation by impairing the intestine's permeability. Those who take these drugs for relief of, say, rheumatoid arthritis, may be making their condition worse in the long run.

Alcohol is absorbed into the blood directly from the stomach and upper small intestine. On its way through, it can destroy cells in the stomach and intestinal linings. Consuming alcohol with food helps to minimize this damage. The healthy body can metabolize small amounts of alcohol; however, anyone with a suspected leaky gut would be wise to avoid alcohol completely.

Candidiasis is an overgrowth of the fungus, *Candida albicans* – which starts in the gut and can then spread to the general circulation. Many people with candidiasis have been heavy users of broad-spectrum antibiotics, steroid drugs, or birth control pills. These drugs destroy the beneficial microflora in the intestines that are the natural antagonists of *C. albicans*.

Food allergies can also weaken the intestinal lining. Allergies attack a particular target organ. If that target happens to be the small intestine, then its lining can be damaged. Some susceptible individuals (including those not sensitive to gluten) may impair their intestinal permeability from consuming such foods as wheat, the nightshades, caffeine, or citrus fruits.

FOOD ALLERGIES

One of the most common symptoms of food allergies is the inflammation they cause in various parts of the body – including joints, pancreas, thyroid, colon, blood vessels, lymph vessels, and the myelin sheath covering nerves. Some conditions considered autoimmune may instead be caused by deeply entrenched food allergies – including rheumatoid arthritis, thyroiditis, ulcerative colitis, and vasculitis.

To find out to what extent hidden allergies may be involved in any disorder, implement meticulously the principles explained in the chapter, "One's Food is Another's Poison", about how to identify and eliminate suspected food allergens. This can be a daunting task and well worth the effort. If total elimination of all food culprits either corrects the condition in question or completely stops its progression, this is proof positive that it was primarily caused by allergies.

Rheumatoid arthritis is a case in point. Its progression can be halted by total elimination of all food allergens. The disfigurement of hands and feet cannot be reversed, but can serve as a pain-free reminder of what was and no longer is. It takes both desire and discipline to eliminate the foods to which one is addicted, and not everyone is ready for that. One lady defiantly told me that she would rather die than give up her sweets – and her wish was granted some painful years later.

A THREE STEP PROGRAM

Not knowing everything about autoimmunity does not prevent us from taking positive action. There are some things we can do.

The following three step program may be capable of halting the progression of some autoimmune disorders. It can also be used as a form of therapeutic diagnosis – i.e., if the person's condition improves, then one or more of these factors must have contributed to it. Even if strengthening these weaknesses does nothing to slow down an autoimmune disorder, the person's health will definitely benefit in other ways.

1. Take digestive enzymes to overcome the digestive weakness.
2. Eliminate all foods to which the person is allergic.
3. Heal the leaky gut.

ARTHRITIS

Arthritis is literally "inflammation of the joints". If you tell your doctor that your joints are sore and swollen – and he says that you have arthritis – that is exactly what you told him. Arthritis is a symptom, not a disease. Inflamed joints can have a number of causes or contributing factors.

ALLERGIC ARTHRITIS

Most cases of arthritis may be caused by hidden food allergies. When the specific allergens are removed from the diet, the arthritic symptoms disappear. Theoretically, any food could cause arthritis in uniquely sensitive individuals; however, there is a pattern. Number one on the list of culprits to suspect is the nightshade family (tomatoes, potatoes, peppers, paprika, eggplant, chili, cayenne, tobacco). In a study of 5,000 arthritic patients, over 70 percent reported gradually increasing relief from aches, pains, and disfigurement simply by eliminating nightshades from their diet.

Allergy and addiction are two sides of the same coin. If there is a food that one constantly craves and cannot do without, it is most probably an allergen. Someone who has a bottle of hot sauce at the ready in her purse will likely see her arthritis disappear when she eliminates all nightshades. Same for someone who eats green peppers fresh out of the garden every day that it is possible and loads up on them at the supermarket at other times. Similarly, someone addicted to toast and jam may have her arthritis disappear when she eliminates wheat and sugar.

OSTEOARTHRITIS

Osteoarthritis is marked by progressive deterioration of cartilage in synovial joints and vertebrae. Although hidden food allergies may not be the ultimate cause, they can certainly be contributing factors. One study found that total elimination of the nightshades over several months often resulted in gradual improvement of osteoarthritis.

As the body ages, its ability to produce certain factors (e.g., stomach acid, thyroid hormones) naturally declines. So it is also with the synovial fluid that lubricates joints, bursae, and tendon sheaths. The nutritional supplements that help the body maintain its production of synovial fluid include **marine lipids**, **glucosamine sulfate**, **chondroitin sulfate**, and **methyl-sulphonyl-methane (MSM)**. **Manganese** (15 mg. daily) contributes to the strength of supporting ligaments. Large amounts of **vitamin C** (4,000 mg. daily) are also required to rebuild joint cartilage. It is a little known fact that sore and tender joints can be symptomatic of scurvy.

In the absence of traumatic injury or abusive manual labor, osteoarthritis of the fingers tends to be moderate and self-limiting. Knuckles become enlarged and nodular, with minimal pain, fingertips may point in slightly different directions – and that is usually as far as it goes. Osteoarthritis of weight bearing joints (hip, knee) can be a different story. Unless corrective measures are taken, joint replacement surgery (arthroplasty) may be required.

RHEUMATOID ARTHRITIS

Rheumatoid arthritis is a chronic and deeply entrenched systemic condition marked by inflammatory changes in joints and related structures that result in crippling deformities. It is commonly considered to be an autoimmune disorder.

Hidden allergies are a major contributor to rheumatoid arthritis. By totally eliminating the offending foods, it is possible to halt the progression of this debilitating condition. Suspect any and all foods that the person consumes daily and feels she cannot do without (e.g., coffee, sugar, wheat, orange juice, potatoes, tomatoes, or whatever). If the person says, "You're not going to take me off my potatoes!" – then you know the primary allergy/addiction that is involved.

GOUT

Gout is an acute form of arthritis caused by abnormally high levels of uric acid in the blood (hyperuricemia) – in those people who have a hereditary predisposition for this condition. Any joint may be affected by gout, but it usually starts in the knee or foot.

People with gout may need to avoid foods that are high in purines such as meats (especially organ meats), seafood, lentils, beans, peas, and soy – or – they may need to eat lots of cherries. Cherries have the ability to reduce hyperuricemia. It doesn't matter if the cherries are fresh, frozen, canned or juiced. In one study, 12 gout patients on a non-restricted diet ate about one pound of fresh or canned cherries daily. Blood uric acid was reduced to normal in all of them. There is evidence that supplementary folic acid and vitamin C may also help to decrease uric acid levels.

MENTAL HEALTH

Although it is generally accepted that mental disorders have psychological or neurological causes, this is not always true. Some behavioral abnormalities are caused or aggravated by nutritional factors. Even when faulty nutrition is not the cause, good nutrition can always help.

Hypoglycemia causes mood swings, anxiety attacks, fits of anger, agitation, crying spells, constant worrying, nervousness, or depression – all of which can also have other causes. Up to 70 percent of blood sugar is required by the brain, as its fuel. Being unable to store glucose (as glycogen) the way muscles do, the brain is thus highly sensitive to drops in blood sugar levels. To find out if hypoglycemia is involved, all it takes is this therapeutic diagnosis: follow the hypoglycemic diet and take adrenal support. If the mental symptoms go away, they had to have been induced by the hypoglycemic state.

Food allergies can cause various tissues in the body to become inflamed or go into spasm. Sometimes the target organ for allergens is the brain, where they can produce symptoms including convulsions, learning disorders, mental confusion, anxiety, panic attacks, behavioral problems, uncontrolled anger, emotional outbursts, dyslexia, crying attacks, nightmares, hallucinations, delusions, or paranoia. Again, the way to find out if food allergies are involved is to do a therapeutic diagnosis: track down and eliminate all possible offending foods. If the person's mental state improves significantly, then hidden food allergies must have been a contributing factor. Some schizophrenics are able to function symptom free using diet as a control rather than drugs. Potentially any food can cause mental symptoms in an unusually sensitive individual. Start the search for problematic foods with those that the person craves and cannot do without. Wheat and sugar are often high on the list of contenders.

Adrenal weakness can produce mental symptoms including: inability to cope with stressful events, prefer being alone, perfectionism, avoiding complaints, ignoring inconveniences, mood swings, tendency to cry easily, difficulty relaxing, emotional exhaustion, feeling overwhelmed, and feeling defeated. Nutrients that support the adrenal glands include vitamin C, pantothenic acid, vitamin B-12, and potassium.

Thyroid weakness can produce mental symptoms including: dislike working under pressure, dislike being watched, difficulty concentrating, easily distracted, depression, irritability, mood swings, or erratic behavior. Nutrients that support the thyroid gland include iodine, selenium, L-tyrosine, L-cysteine, and vitamin B-12.

DEPRESSION

The hopelessness of mental depression usually results from holding back deep feelings one does not feel entitled to have (such as anger or grief). Vitamins B-1, vitamin B-12, vitamin D, folic acid, magnesium, zinc, and/ or iron may be deficient in those who are prone to depression. Regardless of whether the depression is psychological or biochemical, daily doses of **vitamin B-12** (5,000 mcg.) and **magnesium** (500 mg.) can bring significant relief. Vitamin B-12 is best taken as sublingual tablets that dissolve under the tongue, because this vitamin is poorly absorbed through the intestinal tract.

Many people with low thyroid function tend to be depressed, but this may be because the same thinking pattern which induced the hypothyroidism also created the depression. The more a person tells herself thoughts like, "I don't have a life of my own," and "I never get to do what I want to do," the more the body cooperates by slowing down the thyroid, the master gland that regulates metabolism. If you do not believe that your own life matters, then your thyroid follows that lead. Feeling that you are not important to yourself is a depressing thought on its own, with or without hypothyroidism, so it is hard to know which came first – and from a therapeutic perspective, it does not matter. Everyone suffering

NUTRITIONAL SOLUTIONS FOR 88 CONDITIONS

from depression needs to check out the chapter, "The Underdiagnosed Condition".

PHOBIAS

Phobias are deeply ingrained irrational fears, the causes of which have nothing to do with faulty nutrition – although on one occasion I had the opportunity to see if good nutrition might be able to help. In desperation, the parents of an 18-year old boy suffering from agoraphobia asked me to make a house call. For two years their son had been unable to set foot outside their home. They had even bought him a Porsche as an incentive, but he was afraid to take it out of the garage. What this young man had for breakfast was shocking: a sugar frosted cereal to which he heaped on extra sugar, plus a large bottle of cola. What he ate for the rest of the day was no better. Clearly, he had an allergic addiction to sugar. If he had been able to break the addition, would his agoraphobia have diminished? We will never know. He was unwilling to let go of the belief that what he ate had nothing to do with his condition. My conclusion: belief triumphs over nutrition.

PREMATURE AGING

The human body is programmed to wear out. How fast it ages, however, is a variable that is strongly influenced by belief, lifestyle, diet, and nutritional supplements. It is possible to reverse one's biological age in order to feel, act, and look many years younger.

Where there is no genetic or disease component involved, premature aging is the result of nutritional neglect. Our bodies are bombarded with free radicals from the outside (e.g., carbon monoxide fumes, tobacco smoke, air pollution, X-rays, microwaves, cosmic radiation, chlorinated swimming pools, cleaning fluids) – as well as free radicals generated internally from chemically unstable foods (e.g., polyunsaturated oils, rancid fats, chlorinated drinking water, nitrates, nitrites).

Free radicals take their toll over the years, damaging and cross-linking protein tissues, causing wrinkling of the skin, accelerated aging, and contributing to the development of arterial disease, cancer, and cataracts. Brain and arterial tissue are particularly vulnerable to free radical damage. High potency antioxidants both prevent and reverse free radical damage, making the user look and feel younger.

Improved circulation has a rejuvenating effect on the entire body. The **arterial cleansing formula** (described in the chapter, "Unplug the Arteries") not only improves circulation but also floods the body with antioxidants and other factors that can help improve memory, glandular function, and sometimes even increase sexual desire.

As the body ages, it produces progressively less hydrochloric acid and digestive enzymes. As digestive juices decline, so does the body's ability to absorb and utilize nutrients from the diet. Reduced ability to utilize nutrients ensures that the body will continue to decline even further. This vicious cycle can be reversed by supplementing with the **digestive enzyme formula** [*described in the chapter*, "It Begins with Digestion"].

BELIEFS ABOUT AGING

The rate at which our bodies deteriorate is greatly affected by our beliefs about aging. There is a remote tribe in South America that values both running and age. Men in this village do a lot of long distance running, many kilometers at a time. They fully expect athletic skill to continue to improve with age – and for them it does: men in their 60s consistently outperform those in their 20s. At age 64, I took a page from their book, so to speak, by winning a karate tournament at the University of Maine (in over age 35 category).

If you wish your body to become biologically younger, start with your thoughts. Don't think of yourself as having any particular age. Let go of any assumptions you have about your age or the aging process. The "you" that notices things today feels exactly the same as the "you" who noticed things when you were young. It is as if no time has passed. Just go with that feeling.

There is no health problem that is directly caused by one's age. If there were, then everyone the same age would be in exactly the same state of health. Blaming a given condition on age stops one from looking for its true cause (e.g., faulty diet, nutritional deficiencies, allergies, inactivity, stressful lifestyle, free radicals).

A 55-year old gentleman once came to me concerned about muscle wasting. Flesh hung loosely from his left upper arm but was quite firm on his right. When he had asked his doctor what caused this condition, he was told, "It is just your age." I suggested that he ask his doctor why the other arm wasn't affected, since both arms were exactly the same age. A change in diet and supplementary B-complex vitamins had both arms equally firm within six weeks.

We have come to accept wrinkled skin, lower energy, decreased libido, muscle wasting, and forgetfulness as an inevitable part of growing older – but they don't have to be, at least not at the rate that we take for granted. Those who age gracefully usually don't think of themselves as being any particular age and are often surprised at what the numbers reveal when the next birthday rolls around. Healthy seniors believe that they are only as old as they feel, that life is for living, and they enjoy life doing things they consider to be fun.

SKIN CARE

A huge industry profits from creams and lotions intended to reduce wrinkling. The better of these provide antioxidants, vitamins, and moisturizing factors. There is, however, a limit to the kinds of molecules that can be absorbed through the skin, which nature has deliberately intended to be a selective barrier.

The skin is nourished from the inside. To remain healthy and wrinkle-free, it needs vitamin A, Vitamin E, oleic acid, essential fatty acids – and it especially needs vitamin C and protein to form elastin and collagen. Elastin is a protein in connective tissue. Collagen is the "glue" or matrix not only for skin cells but also for those in bone, ligaments and connective tissue.

The skin reflects what is happening inside. Wrinkles on the face and neck indicate that collagen tissue throughout the body is deteriorating faster than it can be replaced. Vitamin C is crucial to the formation of collagen. Smokers develop wrinkles much faster than non-smokers, so much so that the term, "smoker's face" has been coined to describe this phenomenon. Each cigarette smoked depletes the body of about 25 mg. of vitamin C (40 percent of its RDA).

An internal skin restoration program needs to include at least the following daily amounts of supplements: **vitamin C** (4,000 mg.), **vitamin E** (600 I.U.), **vitamin A** (20,000 I.U.), two to three tablespoons of **olive oil** (for its oleic acid content), plus 60 grams of dietary **protein**.

HYDRATION

One of the surer ways to look older than your years is not to drink enough water. The body needs lots of water. It is the medium in which all biochemical reactions take place. It is the medium in which toxins are excreted. It is required in abundance for the health of the kidneys.

Many people are dehydrated without knowing it, for two reasons: (1) by the time one feels thirsty, the body is already dehydrated; and (2) they do not recognize the symptoms of dehydration. These symptoms include:

- □ Dry or leathery skin.
- □ Dry or chapped lips.
- □ Dry mouth.
- □ Dry eyes.

- □ Dry nasal membranes.
- □ Stools hard and dry.
- □ Low volume of urine, urinate infrequently.
- □ Tendency to form kidney stones.

Stay ahead of the game by drinking continually throughout the day. Ideally, each adult needs to consume a minimum of two litres (quarts) of purified water daily. Some of this liquid intake can be in the form of herbal teas, decaffeinated coffee, or dilute unsweetened juices. If, however, caffeinated or alcoholic beverages are consumed, then the amount of purified water needs to be increased accordingly.

EXERCISE

Your body thrives on physical activity. Regular exercise stimulates lymphatic drainage. Lymph fluid (the intermediary between the blood and bodily cells) exchanges nutrients and carries wastes away. There is more lymph than blood, but it must circulate without benefit of a heart or pump. It needs the massage that exercise affords, in order to keep it flowing.

Muscles thrive on the challenges we give them. Exercise tones muscles, eases stress, stimulates internal organs, enlarges blood vessels, relieves depression, promotes sleep, helps to lower cholesterol, and facilitates clear thinking. In other words, exercise is rejuvenating

Light stretching/flexibility exercises performed first thing in the morning, while the spine is relaxed, are reputed to add years to one's life. Tai chi, yoga, or Pilates are ideal for this purpose, as are any warmup movements that emphasize gentle stretching of the long muscles and circular motions of the joints.

Exercising vigorously for 30 minutes at a time, two or three times per week, is especially rejuvenating. Brisk walking, dancing, cycling, treadmill, racquet sports, swimming, aerobics – are all excellent choices. Choose an activity that you enjoy for its own sake, so that the doing of it will be pleasurable rather than a contest of will power.

If your body is fragile, has limited range of motion, or a low tolerance for exercise, move into activities gradually. Start with walking. Find out how far you can walk without undue discomfort. Each day you go out, walk a little further.

REST

Stress ages. The more demands we place on our bodies, the less time they have to recuperate and rebuild. Working, commuting, raising children, keeping house, social outings, shopping, sports – all of these activities have a way of cumulating and taking over our lives, if we let them. If your day is spent rushing from one activity to another with no time left to relax and unwind, you are overtaxing your body, succumbing to what may be called "the hurry sickness". Such undue stress contributes to fatigue, adrenal exhaustion, immune weakness, and bodily degeneration. Stress causes the adrenal glands to shift into a "fight or flight" mode – which operates continually in the background when one is overwhelmed by pressure, fear, anxiety, worrying, or unrelenting mental activity.

However busy your schedule may be, build in 20-minute rest breaks or "power naps", once or twice daily. Sit in nature, listen to soft music, shut your door, hold all calls, or find a private cubicle somewhere. Close your eyes, take a deep breath, and give your mind a complete vacation. Listen to your breathing. Let your thoughts drift wherever they wish, without restraint. Let go completely. At some point your mind will gap out – and when you come to, you will feel calm and refreshed. Notice how much more vivid colors appear and how much more easily you can focus your attention on whatever you wish.

Let go of the notion that if you take a break, you won't have time to do everything you have to do. The mental clarity and rejuvenating effect of a power nap helps you to accomplish more with less effort, and also to see new possibilities for making more efficient use of your time.

It is also very healing and rejuvenating to take one day per week of complete leisure. Seal out the outside world, stay in bed, listen to music, sit or walk in nature, read, watch movies – do whatever you find relaxing and enjoyable, or do nothing in particular.

INDEX TO 88 CONDITIONS

YOU CAN BE YOUR OWN DOCTOR

Most people with chronic health complaints visit their doctors to be prescribed medications that are often taken for life. These have significant side effects and never address the reasons for the illness. Conventional medicine rarely looks into the causes of high blood pressure, diabetes, heart disease, arthritis and cancer. It's as if it doesn't really matter what caused it. But you know it does.

You will find, by reading this treasury of information, answers to why illness develops and natural solutions to reversing 88 chronic health concerns. There is one truism I have learned after 38 years of medical practice: *"For whatever condition a drug is prescribed to treat an illness, there is always a natural remedy that will work just as well or better and with far fewer side effects."* This is something you will also learn from this book. ***You can be your own doctor, and this book will show you how.*** Whatever health challenges are facing you, please read this book before resorting to a lifetime of dangerous drugs and other questionable conventional treatments.

Zoltan P. Rona*, M.D., M.Sc., Holistic Medical Doctor*

ABOUT THE AUTHOR

David Rowland is Canada's foremost expert in holistic nutrition. He is the innovator and publisher of Nutritiapedia®, the free on-line nutritional encyclopedia, as well as being the author of 12 highly acclaimed health publications. David is the creator of the Nutri-Body® assessment method favored by natural health practitioners for determining biochemical weaknesses. He founded the Canadian Nutrition Institute (1983), the Nutritional Consultants Organization of Canada (1983), and the Edison Institute of Nutrition (1996). David is also court recognized as an expert in complementary medicine.

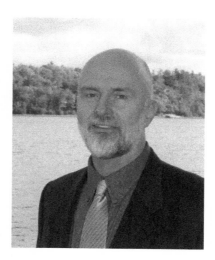

CPSIA information can be obtained
at www.ICGtesting.com
Printed in the USA
LVHW02s0403040518
575768LV00001B/1/P

9 781504 369787